D1044191

SUFFERED LONG ENOUGH

A physician's journey of overcoming
Fibromyalgia, Chronic Fatigue, & Lyme

WILLIAM RAWLS, MD

© 2014 William Rawls, MD

All Rights Reserved.

No part of this publication may be reproduced, stored in a retrieval system, or transmitted, in any form or by any means, electronic, mechanical, photocopying, recording,
or otherwise, without the written permission of the author.

First published by Dog Ear Publishing
4010 W. 86th Street, Ste H
Indianapolis, IN 46268
www.dogearpublishing.net

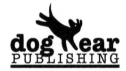

ISBN: 978-1-4575-3069-2

Library of Congress Control Number: 2014953731

This book is printed on acid-free paper.

Printed in the United States of America

Image credit for front cover
© 2014 H. Kopp-Delaney
Some Rights Reserved (Creative Commons License 2.0)
http://www.koppdelaney.de/

CONTENTS

PREFACE

Fatigue is possibly the most common complaint heard in primary care medicine today, and certainly, it is one of the most frustrating complaints that providers have to deal with. Fatigue is common with many diseases, but it is not specific for any disease. There are no drugs that specifically treat fatigue. When fatigue becomes chronic, it is defined as a syndrome, and when it becomes associated with muscle pain at trigger points, it is called fibromyalgia. For patients with chronic fatigue or fibromyalgia, life can be extremely frustrating and sometimes even terrifying; no one understands why you are sick, and no doctor can make you well. For half of my life, I have been one of those patients.

When I was recovering from what I came to know as chronic fatigue/fibromyalgia, I always envisioned myself as having fallen down an old well—the outer stone wall marking the opening being long gone, and the area covered with leaves and debris, making it an easy trap. The circular inner sides of the well were made of flat stones, stacked one on top of another and mortared together; this created crevices where fingers and toes could grasp. There I clung, struggling for my life. Looking up, I could see a tiny round circle of light; looking down, only darkness. It was always cold and damp, and most of the time, except on occasions when the sun was just right, I felt chilled to the bone.

During the day, I would claw my way upward, inch by inch. Some days I would make steady progress, others, not so much. On bad days, I would lose my grip and slip downward several feet before I could rest, recover, and then start back up again. On the worst days, I would fall and barely regain my grip. A few times, I thought how easy it would be just to let go and keep falling, but I never did; I'm not a quitter. At night, I would cling to the walls and sleep uncomfortably, if at all.

It went on like this for years. My predicament was not visible to most people; only a few understood. I am a private person. Initially,

I sought help from conventional medical colleagues, but their efforts actually made my situation more precarious, and drug therapies carried me deeper into darkness. Positive change began to occur only when I shifted my attention toward researching and understanding the causes that had carried me down in the first place.

With a complete change in diet and lifestyle, I began making upward progress, slowly but steadily. The speed of progress increased when I fully embraced natural therapies. My strength returned, and my bodily functions normalized. There were still bad days, but upward progress was more the norm. Finally, I reached the opening...and then promptly fell back in. This happened numerous times before I was truly free.

Standing securely on level ground, there is no celebration; I know the opening will always be close by and that falling back in is a never-ending possibility. Life will never be quite the same; steps will have to be taken carefully. Oddly, however, I gained more than I lost during all those years. I learned about myself. I learned skills that I would have never known otherwise. I discovered my true purpose.

Now I help others who have fallen into old wells. I know that the walls of the well are very fragile—direct intervention could cause catastrophe. Throwing down a rope as a lifeline and shining a light to guide the way is the best that I can offer. By my reducing some of the weight, allowing extra rest, and guiding proper foot and finger holds, maybe that person's climb will not be quite so hard or quite so lonely.

FOREWORD

A LIFE OF CHRONIC FATIGUE

Chronic fatigue is certainly not a life I would have chosen; it chose me. Often, things happen that way. Even as early as grade school, I can remember not having as much oomph as other kids; dead last seemed to be my token position at all sporting events. Stubbornness and perseverance carried me over most of life's obstacles, however, and I was able to get through college, medical school, and a busy residency in Ob/Gyn. During early years in private practice, I was able to balance family life with a busy work schedule. Fatigue was just part of the picture—I thought it was normal. Fatigue did not become a chronic problem until my mid-forties.

By then, I had been taking obstetrics call every third night for almost fifteen years. The long and often odd hours were taxing, and my ability to bounce back finally fizzled completely. Adding new partners to my group and spreading out the call seemed to be a logical solution, but even that was not enough. Getting any sleep on call nights became impossible, and nights off call were not much better. Fatigue with joint and muscle pain became a real issue. I finally sought help at a sleep clinic and came away with a prescription for a sleeping pill. Reluctant, but desperate, I used the pill, which ensured sleep on nights off call. It became my salvation, and everything was better for a while.

The salvation was short lived, however, and sleep continued to deteriorate. Obstetrics call became so oppressive that I was finally forced to give it up completely. Without being able to take call, I was forced to resign from my group. At that point, I probably should have declared disability, but with optimism that recovery was possible, I opened a solo practice in gynecology and primary care. Keeping up with a 9-to-5 schedule and turning over enough patients to pay the bills, however, was an extreme challenge.

Stubbornness was the only thing that kept me going. Insomnia worsened. Fatigue and pain became constant, but fear of narcotics kept me from using anything stronger than ibuprofen. Joints creaked and crunched with every movement. Burning feet were a constant misery. I began having an irregular heartbeat and vague discomfort in my chest. By then, I was completely dependent on the sleep medication, and it was working only marginally. One night, it finally stopped working altogether. Talk about terror. Not sleeping for several nights in a row and knowing that a full day of work was in store the next day was a nightmare of the worst kind. I learned about panic attacks. My internist added medications to help me sleep and to calm me, but it wasn't much of a solution. There was little joy left in life.

To my surprise, an extensive medical evaluation by my internist disclosed nothing of great pertinence. Thyroid function was normal. Fasting blood sugar was up a bit—no surprise, as my dietary habits were nothing to brag about. Blood pressure was also high, but that wasn't a surprise, either, considering the stress; another medication was prescribed to keep it down. A screening test for Lyme disease was negative. Autoimmune disease did not appear to be a factor. Treating symptoms was all my internist had to offer, and the drugs just made me feel worse. Chronic fatigue or fibromyalgia was the only possible diagnosis—and both were diagnoses of exclusion, when nothing else fits.

Neither were diagnoses I wanted. They carry a stigma. Doctors like things they can define and treat. If you have something that is hard to define and has no specific (or easy) treatment, they don't want to mess with it. I knew the feeling. There is nothing worse than walking into an exam room and finding a patient with a two-page list of diffuse symptoms and knowing that you have only fifteen minutes to figure things out—extremely frustrating for patient and provider alike. The most that can happen is a cursory review and prescriptions aimed at symptoms.

Suddenly, that patient was me. Though every provider I came in contact with was polite, I could almost sense them roll their eyes whenever I came through the door.

I had been relying on exercise to achieve brief episodes of feeling normal (endorphins are wonderful!), but my ability to exercise was becoming progressively limited. One exercise was surfing; I couldn't catch waves quite like everyone else, but it felt good just to get out there. One warm fall day, I was out after work. The waves were small and the wind was totally calm: a picture-perfect day. I was the only one out. After only two waves, my heart was beating so irregularly and the chest pain was so intense, I came in to the beach. As I lay on the sand, it seemed like the end. Staring up into the sky, I relaxed my body and waited. With time, however, my heart did settle down. I picked up the board and walked to the car. Nothing left. Exercise had kept me going; now it was gone.

The next day at the internist's office, an EKG showed mild ischemia (decreased oxygen supply to the heart), and the following day, I was at a cardiologist's office, scheduled for cardiac catheterization. The IV was placed improperly, so I had little anesthesia for the procedure—I heard, felt, and saw the whole thing. When the cardiologist talked with me after the procedure, I was already aware that my vessels were clean as a whistle. He offered no explanation for the peculiar behavior of my heart and suggested that I would have to live with it. A prescription for a beta-blocker to inhibit the irregular beats was all that was offered; I could take it if I wanted, or not—my choice.

That was enough. I had experienced the full gamut of conventional medical therapy, and my situation had worsened progressively. All the doctors had to offer was drugs to cover up symptoms, no real cure. Wellness did not seem to be in their vocabulary. It was time for me to take charge. There had to be a reason for my condition; cause and effect is a fundamental law of the universe. Deep inside, I knew if I could restore my own health, I could help many other people do the same.

I poured myself into nutrition textbooks and reviewed updated versions of all the basic medical textbooks. Unlike in medical school, however, my perspective had changed in a critical way. My focus was now on searching for root causes of disease rather than on how to treat disease. Anything and everything I could find in the lay press that might be applicable, I also devoured. Intuition led me to explore natural therapies, where ultimately, I would find many answers. I had harbored an interest in herbs for a long time;

now I immersed myself in the topic, went to conferences, and became certified in holistic medicine.

Everything I learned, I applied to myself. I designed a basic regimen of natural supplements and took them religiously. I had cleaned up my dietary habits completely and was getting stress under control. Fatigue and pain were present, but I could function. Heart palpitations and chest pain had diminished enough to allow low-intensity exercise. I was finally clawing my way upward. My new medical practice became a reflection of everything I learned. Health restoration became the primary theme. Old patients started returning, and new patients were coming in the door every day. As I started climbing out of the hole, my medical practice followed. Work was stressful, but I managed to keep up with the pace.

Things were looking up, but I was still very dependent on the sleep medication and began to appreciate that some of my symptoms might actually be a reaction to that dependence. I found a protocol for benzodiazepine withdrawal (most sleep medications are benzodiazepines or close relatives, and they are the most habituating substances on earth) and got my internist on board to help me out. After a year of hard work, I was successful. Sleep was far from being perfect off the drug, but I could maintain with natural supplements and intermittent use of a non-benzodiazepine drug that helped with sleep.

Other symptoms associated with chronic fatigue were still present but had diminished enough to allow a relatively normal life. I wasn't well, but at the same time, I wasn't getting any worse, either. I learned to cover up my disability; most people were not aware. I was beginning to believe that things would be okay...that is until the "second" tick bite occurred.

It was July, the end of the second year in the new practice. I was feeling pretty good, the best in a while. I had spent a weekend clearing brush for a garden; it felt great to be outdoors, doing physical work. The next week, a strange itchy rash migrated around my whole body. Overall, however, I felt fine. At the end of that week, Sunday morning, to be exact, I scratched off a scab from a chigger bite that I had been nursing on my right buttock. Much to my surprise, the scab had legs; it was a tick! Over the weeks that followed, all the symptoms that I had been fighting for years came back with a vengeance.

Interestingly, the definitive test for Lyme disease, called a western blot, was suggestive, but not absolutely diagnostic, for Lyme disease. That's how it is with most cases of "Lyme disease." I can't absolutely tell you today whether or not I was infected with Borrelia burgdorferi, the bacterium that causes Lyme. These types of microbes are remarkably stealthy. I had most all of the symptoms of Lyme disease, both acutely and chronically, but those symptoms are nonspecific and overlap with other conditions. Also, ticks carry many different types of pathogenic microbes; some, we may not even be aware of yet. I did have a rash around the tick bite that lasted for months, but it never absolutely declared itself as the classic bull's-eye rash (that happens in only a third of cases). I was quite confident, however, of the fact that I was dealing with some type of bacterial infection, and the possibility of Lyme disease could not be excluded.

Antibiotic therapy was indicated, so I again turned back toward the medical establishment for help. About a week into the first antibiotic prescription, my condition started to improve, but by the second week, my very sensitive gastrointestinal system was a mess. I took a break for a couple of weeks and tried again. Same response. I added high doses of probiotics and tried again. And again the same response. The Lyme symptoms improved, but side effects prohibited chronic use of antibiotics.

So, Plan A with conventional antibiotic therapy was not satisfactory; I would have to find other options...but at least, for the first time, I knew what I was dealing with. I call it the "second" tick bite because I had spent much of my youth outdoors and tick bites had been a near daily affair. The possibility that I had been harboring some tick-borne microbe all along, even from childhood, is not unlikely. All the symptoms I had been previously having for years, including the heart condition, could be explained by chronic Lyme disease. And the heart symptoms were still very present. I needed a new plan fast. I had read enough to know that chronic heart involvement with Lyme disease was quite serious.

Fate (God, angels, the Force) was once again pushing me toward natural herbal therapy. Through an Internet search, I happened upon a book, called *Healing Lyme*, by a gifted individual named Stephen Buhner. He had researched natural supplements that might have antimicrobial activity against Borrelia, the primary microbe responsible for Lyme disease. The protocol he offered included a long list of natural supplements, all of which I was familiar with. I had actually taken several of them in the past, but never all together, and certainly never at the very high doses that he was recommending.

Desperate, I took a leap of faith. Within a couple of weeks, I had worked up to a whole handful of capsules several times a day. Unbelievably, there were no side effects. Gastrointestinal function actually improved! Within a month, I started crawling out of the hole. Within three months, I was back where I had been before the second tick bite. Joint pain improved, but most importantly, the chest pain started to ease. It was truly a life-altering experience. My life and my medical practice would never be quite the same again.

Recovery was progressive but slow; it takes time to suppress a hidden microbe (or microbes) and to overcome a lifetime of chronic damage. There were ups and downs; stress tolerance was still an issue but was steadily improving. Travel (which I love) was particularly stressful. I became a real homebody and had to live a fairly isolated existence. Fortunately, my wife was very supportive; I wouldn't have made it through without her. Having one or a few support people who understand the situation is really important.

I developed a great passion for herbal and other natural therapies and immersed myself deeply into the study of those topics. With time, I expanded beyond the Buhner protocol. There are so many wonderful herbs out there; the resources for natural healing are almost unlimited. Potential cures for virtually every disease are very likely already present in plants and other natural substances...we just need to start paying better attention. Fortunately, knowledge of those resources is widely disseminated; we are living in extraordinary times.

It is easy to become complacent when life is going well, and it seemed that whenever complacency set in, something would happen and I would have to become vigilant all over again. Through it all, I came to appreciate, fairly specifically, the unique forces that cause disease. Cause and effect is reality; all disease is the result of cause. Approaching disease from a cause point of view makes finding a specific diagnosis a little less relevant. When I help patients understand and reduce causes of diseases, it doesn't seem to matter which disease processes they are suffering from; wellness is possible. The principles can be applied to any condition.

As for my own situation, every year has brought a higher level of function. The capacity of the human body for self-healing is truly remarkable. My joint health is good, and the chest pain is gone. My exercise capacity has increased to near normal for my age. Setbacks are expected but manageable. Deep in my tissues, hidden microbes are likely still present; maintaining optimal immune function is essential to stay ahead. Taking a handful of carefully chosen supplements twice daily and rotating them regularly is a small price to pay to ensure good health. Maintaining optimal dietary and health habits goes without question. The trade-offs are worth it. I have my life back.

I've read other books describing chronic fatigue as a special journey that will enrich your life, but clinging to the cold damp stone walls of an old well is not a fate I would wish on anyone. It's better to see chronic fatigue for what it is—a chronic debilitating disease process that robs joy from life—and do whatever necessary to get over it as quickly as possible. You may have discovered that the conventional healthcare system really has little to offer; because your condition is poorly understood, the system doesn't really have time or resources to care. And you have probably dabbled with alternative therapies but still not found everything you are looking for. What you need is for someone to put all the pieces together. That is what this book is all about!

INTRODUCTION

OVERVIEW

If the analogy of clinging to the inner walls of a cold damp well accurately describes your present situation, then you are probably ready for a positive change. Making that change, however, requires undoing all the things that landed you in this situation in the first place. Of course, you need to know what those things are. Part I of the book, "Understanding Chronic Fatigue," is devoted to that purpose.

The first chapter of Part I examines fatigue-related disorders and how they are presently viewed by the medical establishment. Chapter 2 goes a little deeper and explores the underlying factors that set the stage for chronic fatigue and related disorders. Chapter 3 gets to the root of the problem by revealing hidden microbes that play a defining role in most fatigue-related disorders. The final chapter of Part I includes a questionnaire and self-assessment for establishing a baseline of your present health.

Part II, "Essential Support," will help you jump-start your recovery. In two separate chapters, supportive therapies—including natural supplements essential to your recovery, certain medications, and acute options for management of pain and sleep—are thoroughly covered. Supportive therapies are designed to reduce symptoms, enhance immune function, and suppress hidden microbes. The benefit is passive; all you have to do is take something.

Supportive therapies can shorten the journey but, alone, will carry you only so far; the complete transformation requires your active participation. Gaining freedom from the cold damp well of fatigue and reaching solid ground requires undoing old habits and learning new habits. The old habits are mostly superficial attachments. Like sandbags tied to your waist, they are weighing you down. Let them go, and the climb automatically gets easier. The new habits are not necessarily unpleasant as compared to what you are doing now (in fact, you may find life to be better all the way

1

around), but they are different...and different requires adjustment. Part III, which includes four chapters, "Nourish," "Purify," "Balance," and "Restore," is devoted to helping you adjust.

The final chapter, "Summary," condenses the entire recovery protocol into a neat and convenient checklist. You can skip over and take a look at it now if you like! You may even want to start following some of the basic recommendations. This will give you a jump start on getting well. Then, sit back, relax, and enjoy reading the book!

How long it takes before your health improves depends on the degree of dysfunction, how long your condition has been present, and how vigorously each component of the protocol is followed. Progress is measured in weeks, months, and years, not days; be patient. The investment, however, is always worth the effort. In most cases, every year will be better than the last. The clock is ticking, and every year that you put off pursuing recovery is another year of living with the misery of chronic fatigue. In contrast, a year spent embracing concepts in this book is a year closer to enjoying a better life!

If you need more help, visit rawlsmd.com and vital-plan.com for recipes, protocols, online consults, and other vital resources.

GETTING INTO THE RIGHT STATE OF MIND

First and foremost, you must take control of your own recovery. Establishing a relationship with a healthcare provider can be beneficial, but you must remain in charge. Be choosy. Ask around. Do an Internet search. Find one who is willing to listen and offer guidance without dictating therapy. Someone who has actually overcome chronic fatigue or who works with chronic fatigue/fibromyalgia patients routinely is the ideal choice. If you have been diagnosed with Lyme disease, finding a provider who understands the complexities of Lyme disease will be to your advantage. The same is true with thyroid disease. A thorough medical evaluation is sometimes indicated to uncover hidden threats that may respond to targeted therapy, but it should not overshadow the need for complete health restoration.

Get extra help if you need it. Hire a health coach. Health coaches guide you through the transformation; they can make the whole process easier. Yoga instructors, physical therapists, chiropractors, and others can also shorten the pathway to wellness. All of these individuals are eager to provide motivation and support.

Go with the flow. Be willing to look at life differently. The lifestyle required for overcoming chronic fatigue is gentle and relaxed. If you are a person used to driving through life, always choosing the most challenging way of getting something done (I was), then prepare for a change. Slow down and live life more deliberately. This journey is about finding your way, not about testing your courage and stamina. Changing your perspective often reveals hidden magic.

Prioritize. From this point on, your entire focus in life should be on getting well. Getting well is more important than job, relationships, friends, food, sports, hobbies, or anything else—because without good health, none of those things really matter. Do not let anything distract you from this goal! The start of each day provides a new opportunity to renew your health!

Learn to say no! Set limits for what you can accomplish in a day; your recovery depends on it. Helping others, social events, and family affairs may have to take a backseat for a while. Be patient; it takes time to learn a new lifestyle, but the reward is getting your life back.

Allow time for recovery. Your recovery depends on down time. Sleep and rest are when the body is in optimal repair mode. Shift your body into repair mode as frequently as possible by allowing plenty of time for rest and sleep.

Do not accept your situation. Acceptance leads to complacency, and complacency leads to stasis. Not moving in a positive direction increases the need for drugs to control symptoms. Work every day to overcome your condition. Anger can be a positive force as long as it doesn't get out of hand; channel it into positive actions instead of negative emotions. Know that overcoming chronic fatigue often opens up greater purpose and meaning in life.

Record your progress. As you change your approach to life, symptoms associated with chronic fatigue will gradually dissipate. The changes, however, are very subtle, and keeping a journal can help you monitor progress. Pick specific symptoms or bodily functions as monitor points. Define these points quantitatively (on a scale of 1–10 if you like), so that change is evident (or not). The questionnaire in Chapter 4 not only is good for establishing your baseline health but also can be used to help you monitor progress.

Avoid focusing on just treating symptoms. Symptom relief is important, but complete recovery is very dependent on restoring normal functions of the body. Drugs can be useful for relieving symptoms, but they have little capacity to restore wellness. Excessive drug use actually impedes recovery.

Natural supplements are the key to getting well. Natural supplements offer advantages of reducing causes of disease and normalizing function. They are a huge part of creating an optimal healing environment within your body. This book discusses natural supplements felt to offer the highest potential for benefit. A knowledgeable healthcare provider can help prioritize supplements and define optimal dosing. Poor response to supplements can often be linked to poor-quality products or inadequate dosing.

Follow your internal GPS. Your intuition is like an internal GPS that guides you through life's journeys. When you veer in the wrong direction, it persistently steers you back to the correct path. When you become completely lost, it plots a whole new course that safely carries you to the destination by a different route. Too often, however, life's distractions prevent us from hearing the voice and we lose our way. Fortunately, the voice of intuition is patient...and there is no greater source of knowledge. Tapping into it is a simple matter of turning down the volume on all the other distractions and paying attention!

A NOTE TO SIGNIFICANT OTHERS

Chronic fatigue/fibromyalgia definitely strains relationships. You may not be feeling the pain, but you are definitely living the misery. Constantly being around someone in ill health is nothing short of exasperating. And because you are the only one who really under-stands the situation, you often receive the brunt of the complaints. Remember, the person suffering has little control over the way he or she feels. Even though on the outside he or she may look pretty normal, inside, that person may feel terrible. Imagine how you feel on the worst day of having the flu, and then imagine feeling that way all the time.

The best thing you can do is give your loved one support when he or she asks for it and give him or her space when support is not requested. Encourage your loved one to help him- or herself when-ever possible; you don't want to create dependence. Sometimes that person may need to sleep in a separate room to get a good night's sleep; it's not personal.

Live for the good times, and tolerate the rest. Allow room, and give support for doing the things necessary to restore health. If you partner in this endeavor, your health will benefit also. Be sure to take time and space for yourself. Living with a person in a debili-tated state can drain your energy; you need to be able to restore.

DISCLAIMERS AND DISCLOSURES

Following the advice in this book offers no guarantee of a cure. No clinical studies have been done specifically on the recommenda-tions discussed. Many patients, however, have gained remarkable benefit from following the advice offered. Though the total protocol has not been evaluated by clinical study (from a practical point of view, it probably never will be), all the information discussed is backed by good solid science. Possibly more importantly, it is backed by logical conclusions based on sound science (science is very dependent on logic and only works if the two are paired).

The risk of potential harm from following any of the advice in this book is remarkably low. The advice in this book is not meant to replace a relationship with a qualified healthcare provider; in fact, it is meant to complement that relationship. Here is the standard disclaimer: The advice offered in this book is not meant to diagnose, treat, or cure any disease.

Therapies exist that are not discussed here that could potentially offer benefit. My passion is herbal therapy, and my training was in surgery and drugs, so therein lies my greatest expertise and the focus of this book. Having a strong background in science restricts my scope primarily to therapies that can be explained by mainstream science. Alternative therapies mentioned either have good science to back them up, such as acupuncture, or have very low potential for harm, such as energy medicine.

I'd like to disclose that I am affiliated with a supplement company, Vital Plan, that I founded with my daughter in 2009. Wading through marketing hype to find only substandard products used to be a constant frustration in my medical practice. Realizing this, my daughter made the career jump to oversee the development of a supplement company where we could control quality and proper dosing. Over the years, we have connected with an incredible team of healthcare providers who have joined our mission to help patients reduce causes of disease through natural supplements and lifestyle changes. I have received invaluable feedback from these providers and their patients that has greatly furthered my efforts to develop innovative wellness solutions at Vital Plan.

Through the company, we have put together combinations of supplements that meet the specifications of this book. If you are interested, you can access them through the Vital Plan website. That being said, this book is meant to provide information, not to be a marketing tool. All natural therapies discussed in this book are referred to very generically and can be obtained from multiple sources.

PART ONE

UNDERSTANDING CHRONIC FATIGUE/FIBROMYALGIA

Here you are, reading yet another book on chronic fatigue…or possibly this is your first. Either way, like so many frustrated individuals, you are searching for answers. You want to know how to free yourself from the misery of chronic fatigue. Likely, so far your focus has been primarily on treating symptoms. And no doubt, part of the reason you are here is because that approach has not been entirely successful. Treating symptoms alone is putting the cart before the horse. To solve the problem of chronic fatigue, you must understand what causes chronic fatigue. For such a misunderstood disease, that can be a tall order—but it is possible.

This first section of the book is devoted to helping you better understand what is going on inside your body. You are not defective. Likely, you can remember a time when you were healthy, and you can be that way again. Right now, however, your body is caught in a tailspin, and the specific factors and circumstances that came together to cause that tailspin must be identified and reversed. It is the key to getting well.

CHAPTER 1

OUTDATED
TWENTIETH-CENTURY SOLUTIONS

By now, you've probably been to see one or more doctors. You may have taken the medications inevitably offered...anything to make the discomfort go away. But you have probably already discovered that even though medicines can give you brief respite from the misery, drugs alone have little capacity to provide a cure.

In the absence of a cure, at least knowing a reason for the suffering would be comforting, but even that has been a disappointment. Tests have been run, and nothing significant ever shows up. Likely, your thyroid is normal (though you may have many symptoms of low thyroid[1]). Cholesterol and blood glucose may be mildly elevated (especially if you are over forty), and your white blood cell count may be on the low side, but nothing to define a treatable diagnosis. Some exotic autoimmune disease would have been acceptable (at least something to talk about), but no, you have had to settle for chronic fatigue or fibromyalgia...because nothing else fits.

Fatigue is an indication that the body has been stressed in some way; it is associated with virtually every chronic disease process. Sometimes fatigue can be traced to a specific initiating event, a bad flu, trauma such as an automobile accident, a tick bite, extreme emotional trauma, exposure to toxic mold, or even a bad sunburn. Sometimes the cause is not as obvious and fatigue comes

---

[1] Thyroid function is usually the first thing checked, but thyroid function is often normal in patients with fatigue as a primary complaint. Even when thyroid function is found to be low, the abnormal thyroid function is actually not the root cause of the problem. Thyroid dysfunction is the result of specific causes, and though treating the patient with thyroid hormone often helps with symptoms, it does not address the underlying causes. Interestingly, thyroid dysfunction and chronic fatigue share root causes; therefore, it should not be surprising to find they share many common symptoms. Abnormal thyroid function and how it relates to fatigue will be thoroughly covered in Chapter 9, "Balance."

on gradually and insidiously. If an initial stress is not severe and general health is good, the body gradually recovers and life returns to normal. If the healing systems of the body have been compromised, however, the body is left in a state of chronic dysfunction. When a specific disease process cannot be defined, the condition is designated as **chronic fatigue syndrome (CFS).**

Severe fatigue unrelieved by rest is the most defining factor of CFS. Other specific criteria for chronic fatigue syndrome includes general intolerance to any type of stress, muscle weakness and pain, joint pain, ligament pain, mental dysfunction (brain fog), nervous conditions, frequent infections, recurrent flu-like symptoms, low-grade temperature, increased thirst, headaches, paresthesia (burning and tingling in feet and hands), poor sleep, allergic reactions, weight loss, sore throat, swollen lymph nodes, gastrointestinal complaints, and anxiety/depression (who wouldn't be depressed when you always feel like you have the flu?). Sleep disturbances and post-exertion fatigue (exercise makes fatigue worse) are almost always associated with CFS. Symptoms typically wax and wane for years, and acute flare-ups that last for weeks are common. Chronic fatigue is more common in women but certainly is not exclusive to women.

Closely related to chronic fatigue syndrome is **fibromyalgia syndrome (FMS).** Fibromyalgia shares many of the same symptoms but includes chronic pain at specific muscle and tendon locations called trigger points. Trigger points are found at different locations around the body and can be similarly reproduced in different patients. The defining difference between chronic fatigue syndrome and fibromyalgia is the level of pain.

The Naming Game

The terms *chronic fatigue syndrome* and *fibromyalgia* are diagnoses. A diagnosis is simply a way of describing a disease process: a label, nothing more. In the cases of both chronic fatigue syndrome and fibromyalgia, a collection of symptoms defines the diagnosis; the range of symptoms is quite broad and not specific for any disease.

Though experts try to define chronic fatigue syndrome and fibromyalgia as separate entities, the margins between the two often blur. For convenience in this text, I've lumped the two terms into one: chronic fatigue/fibromyalgia syndrome (CF/FMS).

Beyond that confusion, CF/FMS shares many symptoms with other chronic diseases, including autoimmune diseases (rheumatoid arthritis, multiple sclerosis, Sjogren's syndrome, and others) and Lyme disease. And don't forget all the other names commonly used for fatigue syndromes, including Gulf War illness, adrenal fatigue, chronic fatigue and immune dysfunction syndrome (CFIDS), mixed connective tissue disorder, and, not to be left out, myalgic encephalomyelitis (ME)—very frustrating for everyone involved. Even worse, chronic fatigue can be associated with many other symptoms but not fit *any* criteria; not having a diagnosis is the absolute worst situation of all!

In conventional medicine, you need a diagnosis to receive treatment. Doctors always prefer diagnoses that are straightforward and concrete. A patient walks in with a sore throat and has a positive test for streptococcus; with a shot of penicillin, she or he is well in a couple of days. Another has a broken arm, the diagnosis confirmed by x-ray; the bone is set, placed in a cast, and the patient is on the way to recovery. Simple cause and effect: very specific therapy targeted at rectifying the underlying cause. All doctors love practicing this kind of medicine. (Who wouldn't? It's very satisfying when patients always get well!) There's not much satisfaction in treating chronic fatigue, however; the symptom profile is complex, the diagnosis is hard to define, and patients rarely get well...at least with the current approach.

Where We Have Come From

A hundred years ago, the diagnoses of chronic fatigue syndrome and fibromyalgia did not even exist. In 1900, the average life expectancy was age 45, and fear of communicable diseases (plague, cholera, TB, smallpox, malaria, and others) outweighed all other concerns. In fact, most people succumbed to infections or trauma long before chronic disease set in. Advances in medical science in the first half of the twentieth century, however, changed everything.

The ancient perception of "evil humors" as a cause of disease gave way to new and effective treatments targeted at specific causative microbes. Improved public health standards, vaccines, and antibiotics dramatically reduced morbidity and mortality, and the United States set an example for the entire world to follow. It was a heady time for the pharmaceutical industry; life expectancy soared, and many had faith that someday, someone in a lab would find the cure for every disease, even cancer. How we approach disease today was very much defined during that era.

Things have changed a lot since the 1950s, however. Chronic degenerative diseases (heart disease, arthritis, diabetes, cancer, etc.) have mostly replaced deadly communicable diseases (except in third-world countries, where these diseases still thrive). These new-age diseases do not fit the "identify, target, and eliminate" approach that worked so well in the past. Present-day drug therapies focus mainly on controlling symptoms and interrupting the processes of disease, not on treating the underlying cause. With this approach, the outcome of "cure" is less likely and the patient remains in a state of "managed illness." Today, managed illness has become the new norm. People are living longer, for sure, but they are getting sick earlier in life and then living with disease...and doctors' offices and hospitals stay full of patients as a result.

CF/FMS is a diagnosis defined exclusively by symptoms; therefore, conventional therapy targets treating symptoms alone. Because there are so many symptoms, many drugs are often prescribed. Each drug brings with it the potential for toxicity and side effects. When multiple drugs are used to treat CF/FMS, distinguishing between symptoms caused by the disease and symptoms associated with drug side effects is often a challenge. Though treatment of symptoms with drug therapy can be beneficial, when drug therapy is the only therapy, the patient rarely gets well and usually becomes progressively more ill. Sooner or later, CF/FMS progresses to a "real" diagnosis such as rheumatoid arthritis, multiple sclerosis, or some other autoimmune disease...and then the drug therapy really gets toxic.

Where We Are Headed

It's really a matter of perspective. You can look at something from one angle and feel confident that you know it, then turn it around to another angle and it looks totally different. That's the way it is with diseases like CF/FMS. Conventional doctors look at chronic disease from the perspective of symptoms and diagnosis. Looking from that angle, drug therapy looks like the absolute best solution. Our entire healthcare system is based on that view and has been for a long time. But turn it to a different angle and look at disease from the perspective of underlying causes, and the best solutions look quite different. There *are* reasons for your misery, and the root causes of CF/FMS *can* be defined. This knowledge is the key to piecing together the story of CF/FMS.

That story begins with a healthy body. Most every life starts that way. Gradually, over an interval defined as a lifetime, a young, healthy body gives way to a body that can no longer sustain life. What happens during that interval matters. You have a lot more control than you realize.

In fact, about the only thing you have no control over is your genes. You inherited a unique set of genes that are unchangeable. Your genes define many things about you, including your risk for different diseases, but genes alone do not define whether you will get sick from those diseases (for CF/FMS, genetics really plays only a minor role). Other factors beyond your genes matter more...and these factors are quite modifiable.

It all relates to how your body interacts with the surrounding environment. Life does not occur in a bubble, and interaction with the surrounding environment is both mandatory and continual; you can't escape it. Some of the factors that contribute to disease are obvious—poor diet, stress, lack of sleep—and others less so. They add up to compromise the healing systems of the body. Eventually, damage accumulates that can be defined as disease and aging. The type (or types) of disease that occurs depends on genetic risk and how the different environmental factors fall together.

The twentieth-century medical model is not the answer for CF/FMS; science is important, but logic must guide the questions. A twenty-first–century solution must go beyond drugs. Taking advantage of all resources, including the world's vast knowledge of natural therapies, is central to the solution. And, most importantly, you, the patient, must take an active role in the recovery process.

CHAPTER 2

SETTING THE STAGE FOR CHRONIC DISEASE

E verything that happens in the physical universe is the result of cause. We use science to investigate and understand why things happen, including the occurrence of disease. What we know today about disease is vastly superior to what we knew 2000 years ago, or 200 years ago, or actually even 20 years ago. Science, however, is never complete. There are always holes in the knowledge accumulated. Even today, we don't know everything about the human body, and we certainly don't know everything about disease.

Logic is the broader understanding of how things work in the physical universe. It is dependent on knowledge accumulated by science but is not limited by science. In other words, logic can fill in the gaps of things we don't know. Using logic, we can take what we do know and make reasonable conclusions without knowing everything. Logical conclusions evolve rapidly as knowledge increases.

One of the problems of medicine today is absolute reliance on pure science—it's commonly called evidence-based medicine. Proponents of evidence-based medicine base all conclusions about treating disease strictly on scientific evidence alone—logic really plays a very minor role. Because science is never absolute and never all-inclusive, evidence-based medicine is often very limited in scope. It can even lead to erroneous conclusions. Generating scientific evidence takes lots of time; therefore, evidence-based medicine evolves extremely slowly. Because there are so many gaps in understanding diseases like CF/FMS, conventional medicine has not accumulated enough evidence to treat them properly.

Conventional medicine will eventually get there, but it might take a while. We're not going to wait. Instead, we are going to take all the science known at this time and piece it together into a logical explanation of why CF/FMS occurs. With a logical explanation in place, we can start finding reasonable solutions for overcoming CF/FMS. Because of the Internet and the explosion of information that has occurred over the past 20 years, completing that task is easier than ever before. Even with the vast knowledge available, however, there are still gaps to be filled in. Logic will help us fill in those gaps until science catches up. As new science is added, our ability to treat CF/FMS will sharpen even further.

CF/FMS is best explained by breaking things down into smaller topics. Our discussion leads off with genetics. Your genes are the hand that life deals you; how that hand plays out is determined by your interaction with the physical world around you. The discussion continues with six categories of factors that I call system disruptors. System disruptors are environmental factors that adversely affect the chemistry of your body. They disrupt hormonal pathways, cause direct tissue damage, contribute to thyroid and adrenal imbalances, compromise immune function, inhibit the healing systems of the body, and set the stage for CF/FMS (and most other diseases) to occur.

Compromised immune function opens the door to chronic infections with specific types of microbes that define CF/FMS. The ultimate opportunists, they are the real root of CF/FMS. The next chapter is devoted to defining these stealthy threats.

THE REMARKABLE HUMAN GENOME

Forty-six chromosomes, bound together by proteins and encapsulated within a nuclear membrane, are present in every cell in your body (with the exception of red blood cells, which have no nucleus). The genes (DNA) held within those chromosomes provide the blueprint for creating an intact human body, yours slightly different than all others. Those genes also hold the history of the human species, everything your ancestors encountered through time. All of the adaptations to a changing world are recorded. What sometimes seem like defects or limitations in the modern world may actually have been adaptations that allowed your distant relatives to survive in a different world long past.

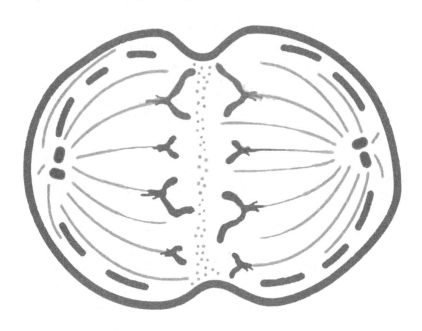

The process of combining chromosomes, an equal share from each of your parents, results in your uniqueness; you are different from all other people, past and present (unless your sibling happens to be an identical twin). You have inherited adaptations from each parent, but you are, of course, not exactly like either parent. And your risks of acquiring different diseases will also not be exactly the same as for either parent or anyone else; no two people carry exactly the same risk for disease. Having risk, however, does not absolutely determine that you will get sick. Genes set the stage, but environmental factors (things you are exposed to) write the script; good health habits can overcome "bad genes."

Fortunately, bad genes and true genetic diseases are relatively rare and account for only 1–2% of all diseases. In the case of CF/FMS, specific genetic factors have not been identified. In other words, you did not directly inherit chronic fatigue from your parents. You may have inherited certain genetic tendencies for both CF/FMS and autoimmune disease from somewhere in your genetic tree—if you happen to be female, your risk is four times greater than if you are male—but these factors are really fairly minor. What is most important is that you do not have a genetic disorder that will prevent you from getting well. Environmental factors play a much larger role—all of which can be modified in your favor!

SYSTEM DISRUPTOR #1: POOR NUTRITION

On the next trip to your local grocery, allow time to take a good look around. Really explore the place. Take stock of all the food and the way it is presented. Once you venture past the produce aisles, the majority of what you will find has been artificially manipulated in some way. The food industry long ago learned that selling packaged and processed food products is much easier and more lucrative than selling fresh food.

Chiefly derived from wheat, corn, and soybeans, these processed food products are specifically designed to touch all human food cravings. They show up on grocery store shelves in attractive and inviting packages, all designed to capture your attention and provide ultimate convenience. (Just throw it in a microwave, and dinner's ready!) Packaged meals, breakfast cereals, bread products, cookies, crackers, and chips account for at least half (50%) the food found in an average grocery store. Other canned and processed foods and grocery store meat comprise another 25%.

Admittedly, these homogenous mixes of processed ingredients are hard to resist. That donut may call out to you every time you pass by, but unfortunately, your body is just not designed to withstand the abnormal concentrations of sugar and starch it contains. Eating these

---

[2] Glucose is the primary fuel for the brain and muscles; blood levels must be constant. When carbs are consumed, a flood of glucose hits the bloodstream. Insulin allows glucose to be taken up by cells, thus lowering blood glucose levels back to normal. Excessive carbohydrate consumption requires excessive insulin secretion. Eventually, cells become resistant to the effects of insulin, and a vicious cycle is created, requiring even higher levels of insulin secretion. The insulin-secreting cells of the pancreas eventually burn out, and blood glucose levels start to rise, signaling the onset of Type II diabetes. Sustained elevated insulin levels are associated with immunosuppression, hormonal imbalance, and promotion of cancer. Glucose causes damage by sticking to proteins throughout the body, compromising function. It also causes cross-linking between strands of molecules such as collagen. Cross-linking accelerates aging and contributes to all disease processes.

types of carbohydrate-rich processed food products damages your tissues directly and causes a state of excess insulin secretion called insulin resistance.[2] Insulin resistance disrupts hormone systems and suppresses immune function. This disruption of body chemistry not only causes fatigue but also sets the stage for CF/FMS. If carbohydrate-rich foods are an everyday habit, sooner or later, diabetes is inevitable.

Excessive starch and sugar are not the only problems associated with processed food products. These types of products also tend to be laden with refined fats. Most people think of fat only as an energy source, but fats (fatty acids) have many important functions in the body. From use as important chemical messengers to making up the cell membranes of every cell in your body, fats are essential. Saturate your body with "bad" fats, and nothing works properly.

Another source of "bad" fat is grocery store meat products. Livestock (poultry, beef, pork) are typically fed an unnatural diet consisting mostly of corn and soybeans. The sole purpose is fattening up the animal as quickly, efficiently, and cost-effectively as possible; neither your health nor the animal's health is a concern. Regular consumption of abnormal fats from artificially fattened meat or processed food products promotes inflammation. Inflammation is the driving force for the pain you may be feeling in your joints and muscles right now. It is also a primary driving force of cardiovascular disease.

All systems of your body are affected by consuming artificially processed food, but your digestive system is especially hard hit. Regular consumption of processed food and fast food inhibits digestion—the body just can't handle these unnatural foods. Everything backs up into your stomach, and esophageal reflux is the inevitable result. Food festers in the stomach, creating a breeding ground for abnormal bacteria such as H. pylori and setting the stage for ulcers. Throw in some everyday stress and you're in real trouble—it's going to take a lot more than Tums or Pepcid to make you well!

Bile, secreted by your liver and stored in your gallbladder, is essential for digesting fat, flushing toxins, and ridding your body of excess cholesterol. Sluggish bile flow, ubiquitously associated with processed food consumption, leads to toxin overload, elevated cholesterol, and gall stones. Starch and sugar also encourage growth of abnormal bacteria and yeast in the gut—gas, bloating, and alternating loose stools and constipation become a normal state. Resulting damage to the lining of the intestines allows foreign proteins from food to "leak" across the intestinal barrier and stimulate the immune system. Hyper-stimulation of the immune system contributes to food sensitivities[3] and immune dysfunction, almost universally present in CF/FMS.

Only the remaining 25% found in the grocery store fits the definition of real food: fresh vegetables and fruit, nuts and beans, whole grains such as oats and brown rice, wild-caught seafood, naturally produced meat, farm-raised eggs, and cold-pressed oils. These foods offer more than just caloric value; they provide vital nutrients that enrich life and the healing capacity of the body. We are actually fortunate to have this 25%. A hundred years ago, fresh foods were available only intermittently in small quantities. Today, because of modern distribution systems, real foods are readily found in most every grocery store across the country. If you are really serious about overcoming CF/FMS, this 25% must become your 100%!

SYSTEM DISRUPTOR #2: EMOTIONAL STRESS

Imagine a primitive human 20,000 years ago sitting in the bushes and eating berries and plant material. His days are defined by the passage of the sun; he has no schedule and no clock. By necessity, he lives in the

---

[3] Allergies to specific foods and sensitivities to food are often used synonymously, but they are not the same. Food sensitivities are associated with immune dysfunction and gastrointestinal dysfunction (caused by stress and eating processed food). Poorly digested proteins from commonly eaten foods "leak" across damaged intestinal barriers and induce immune reactions. Unlike symptoms of true allergy, which are immediate, symptoms of food sensitivities are highly variable, nonspecific, and generally delayed for hours or even days from the time the food is consumed; fatigue is a very common complaint. Typically, multiple foods are involved. Food sensitivities are commonly associated with CF/FMS. Occasionally, food sensitivities are the primary cause of CF/FMS. Generally, food sensitivities will resolve with improvement in health habits and temporary avoidance of offending foods.

moment, every moment. He is not aware of anything outside of his line of sight. Even if lethal threats are close by, presently, they are not his concern. His digestive system is humming along, digesting the food he is consuming. His immune system is functioning optimally, as are other maintenance functions in his body.

It just so happens, however, that there is a lethal threat just around the corner. A roar alerts his attention to a saber-toothed tiger coming his way. At that specific instant, all the resources in his body shift toward escaping that threat. His heart rate speeds up, his vision becomes acute, and his reflexes quicken. His body mobilizes glucose to supply energy for increased muscle activity (blood sugar goes up). The blood inside his blood vessels clots more readily (in case he was slashed by the tiger). In short, he experiences the classic fight-or-flight response. Everyday maintenance functions, including digestive function and immune function, are temporarily placed on hold.

Fortunately, our primitive man performs the correct response—he runs away. Not only does he escape the tiger (this time), but by running, he also normalizes blood pressure and uses up all the mobilized glucose. Everything returns to baseline, and he goes back to eating berries and digesting food. Because he has successfully escaped the tiger, this brief episode of stress has no untoward effect on his body. In fact, the stimulation and exercise probably did him good.

In the modern world, escaping the tiger is an every-minute-of-the-day affair. We are constantly aware of threats not only from around the corner but also from around the globe, many of which are not even real threats—and we do not run from stress but sit and stew about it, worsening the overall effect. A baseline level of chronic stress is much more prevalent than most people realize or accept. The cumulative result can be devastating: elevated blood pressure, increased platelet aggregation (increased blood clotting), compromised digestive function, elevated blood sugar, chronic sleep disturbances, weight gain, and especially suppressed immune function. Uncontrolled stress sets the stage for all diseases...especially CF/FMS.

A little stress is okay; it gets you off the couch and gets you moving. It's the continual unrelenting stress that causes your body to break down. Periodic escape is essential for normal health. There are plenty of ways to do it. Some people turn to meditation and yoga. Others simply learn how to turn it off. What is stressful for one person is pleasurable for another. Regular exercise is a great way to diffuse the detrimental effects of stress. Beyond managing stress directly, you can help normalize the negative physiologic effects of stress with natural supplements.

SYSTEM DISRUPTOR #3: OXIDATIVE STRESS

Right now, inside each and every one of the trillions of cells that make up your body, a fire is burning. It is the fire of life. Though the fire in each cell is infinitesimally small, the flames are intense. The warm glow that is you is a collective reflection of all the fires burning inside your cells. This fire is created by a chemical reaction that generates energy—energy that is essential for life. All functions that occur inside each cell are propelled by energy, but the fire generated must be carefully contained and controlled; the energy unleashed can be destructive. Sparks produced by cellular fire pop off in every direction and have the potential to damage all parts of the cell, including DNA. These sparks are called free radicals[4]...and they are as threatening as the name implies.

---

[4] Technically, free radicals are molecules that steal electrons from other molecules. This process, called oxidation, is the driving force for energy production inside cells, but if not contained, the process is destructive. The primary players are potent free radicals called reactive oxygen species (derived from oxygen). Confining these substances to the reaction site is impossible, and other molecules in the cell, including proteins and strands of DNA, become random targets. Portions of molecules that are affected by oxidation become very reactive, or sticky, and randomly stick to other molecules, a process called cross-linking. Cross-linking renders proteins nonfunctional, and cross-linked DNA strands are the basis for gene mutations that can lead to cancer.

If it were not for chemical compounds called antioxidants, the cell would quickly be consumed by free radicals and the life of the cell would be extinguished. Antioxidants capture and contain free radicals, absorbing the excess energy before it can do harm—cooling the reaction down and restoring balance. Antioxidants are as important for life as is the energy that allows life. Each cell continually creates antioxidant substances internally, but this is never enough. All of your cells also depend on antioxidants that come from things you eat, chiefly vegetables and fruit.

Antioxidants reduce but do not completely eliminate free-radical damage. The net damage caused by free radicals beyond that controlled by antioxidants is called oxidative stress. Of course, the higher the concentration of antioxidants, the slower the rate of damage and the lower the oxidative stress.

Free radicals > antioxidants = oxidative stress.

Oxidative stress is the most basic and fundamental force causing aging and disease. *All* life-forms must deal with oxidative stress, and *all disease processes* have links to oxidative stress. It is most certainly an underlying factor in chronic fatigue. There are three primary sources of oxidative stress: energy production inside cells, inflammation, and toxic substances.

Oxidative stress is as much a part of life as breathing, but the burden of oxidative stress can be influenced by choice of diet and natural supplements. Antioxidants found in fresh vegetables and fruit can certainly tip the balance in a positive direction. Many types of natural supplements can provide antioxidant protection that complements a healthful diet.

Cellular Energy Production

Energy is generated inside cells within microscopic football-shaped structures called mitochondria. Mitochondria are the power source for all cellular functions (imagine miniature power generators churning

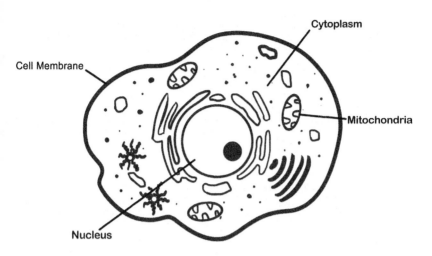

red-hot, with sparks flying). Food molecules are the fuel for the reaction. Adding oxygen to the mix creates an explosion of energy and the free radicals that come with the process. Free radicals radiate outward from mitochondria and have potential to damage all cellular structures, including the DNA that makes up your genes. Free-radical damage unchecked by adequate levels of antioxidants compromises cellular functions and leads to premature cell death (or mutation into a cancerous cell if DNA is severely damaged). This type of oxidative stress is a primary underlying force in aging and all disease.

Of all the vital components inside cells, mitochondria receive the brunt of free-radical exposure—for the mitochondria, generation of energy is a self-destructive process. The resulting damage compromises the ability of mitochondria to produce energy and is central to energy loss (fatigue, muscle weakness) that occurs with CF/FMS. Oxidative stress, however, is not the only threat to mitochondria; certain pathogenic bacteria readily scavenge mitochondria as an energy source. Maintaining optimal protection of your mitochondria is essential for overcoming fatigue associated with CF/FMS.

Antioxidants are essential for limiting cellular damage. Cells generate some antioxidants but also heavily depend on external sources of antioxidants for damage control. Cellular antioxidants can be enhanced with supplemental vitamin C, vitamin E, alpha lipoic acid, n-acetyl cysteine (NAC), and glutathione supplements.

Tissue/Vascular Inflammation

Microbes and other foreign substances are continually gaining entry into your body (it's happening right now in your lungs, skin, and digestive tract). White blood cells, always standing guard, actually produce free radicals to destroy foreign invaders and foreign substances. White blood cells are also responsible for cleaning up waste material and removing dead or dying cells. In addition to producing free radicals, certain white blood cells produce hypochlorous acid and enzymes to break down debris and to expedite the cleanup process.

When this process is kept in balance by antioxidants and other components of the immune system, tissues are protected and positive healing occurs. When the immune system is overwhelmed, tissue damage occurs. This type of damage is called inflammation. Inflammation is one of the primary processes of disease and is also the driving force for pain that occurs in CF/FMS. As mentioned previously, processed food products promote excessive inflammation in the body. Also, as you will learn later, certain microbes actually induce inflammation to break down tissues and scavenge resources. (Your mitochondria are prime targets!)

High consumption of vegetables and fruit reduces inflammation in the body, whereas processed grains, meat, and dairy induce inflammation. Most herbal supplements provide anti-inflammatory properties. Omega-3s (fish oil, flaxseed oil) also balance the inflammatory response.

Oxidative Stress from Toxic Substances

Your body is continually exposed to toxic substances. You depend on your liver to detoxify these substances. The process of detoxification is actually quite toxic—high concentrations of free radicals are produced, and oxidative stress is a greater force in the liver than in any other organ in the body. Throughout a lifetime, your liver takes a quite a beating, and liver cells must be continually replaced. If the ability of the liver to produce new cells is exceeded, fat cells are substituted for liver cells. To some extent, this happens in everyone, and gradual decline in liver function is one reason why risk of disease increases with age. If destruction of liver cells is excessive, however, "fatty liver" results and the processes of aging and disease are dramatically accelerated.

Food can also be a source of free radicals. That chili cheeseburger with fries that may have tempted you yesterday is a deadly combination. Processed oil found in fried food and processed food products is loaded with oxidized fats (oils) that are potent free radicals. These types of free radicals (oxidized polyunsaturated fats) can set off highly destructive chain reactions within your cell membranes. Healthy cell membranes are vital for normally functioning cells and mitochondria. Degradation of cell and mitochondrial membranes certainly contributes to CF/FMS.

Taking good care of your liver is essential for overcoming CF/FMS (and for slowing the aging process). Reducing your toxin load is a great place to start! The herb known as milk thistle is well known for its ability to protect the liver and to actually encourage regeneration of liver cells. Avoiding processed fats and regularly consuming healthful fats (such as olive oil or sesame oil) is great for your liver and your cell membranes. Taking omega-3 fatty acid supplements is another way to protect your cell membranes.

SYSTEM DISRUPTOR #4: TOXIC STRESS

Over the past hundred years, the environment has gradually become saturated in toxic substances, most of which are petroleum-derived. The list of man-made chemicals that are potentially toxic to living things may be as high as 200,000! Beyond all the man-made toxins, mining and burning coal have released an unprecedented amount of heavy metals (aluminum, antimony, beryllium, bismuth, cadmium, lead, mercury, thallium, uranium) into the environment. Toxic substances can even be generated inside your body; consuming processed food contributes to overgrowth of "bad" bacteria, which release toxins that can make you feel terrible!

Though concentrations of specific toxins are rarely high enough to be implicated as causing specific diseases, to think that environmental toxins have no effect on the incidence of disease and cancer would be simple denial of the facts. Toxin accumulation definitely inhibits immune function and certainly plays a central role in CF/FMS.

The technical term for a chemical compound that is toxic to the human body is *xenobiotic*. The list of ways that xenobiotics can adversely affect normal biologic processes is extensive (don't get caught up in the details—just recognize that many types of toxins contribute to disease in a variety of different ways and set the stage for CF/FMS):

- Bond chemically with large molecules (DNA, RNA, proteins), causing direct cellular injury and possible cell death.

- Inhibit normal enzymatic processes in the body directly.

- Damage cell membranes (cell membranes are really important for many normal functions in the body).

- Bind to proteins, altering the way the immune system recognizes itself (this may be one mechanism of autoimmune disease).

- Cause reactions with DNA or directly damage DNA—possibly an initiating factor of cancer.

- Damage liver and kidneys, the primary organs responsible for removing toxins.

- Inhibit normal immune function—especially pertinent to CF/FMS.

- Create free radicals or act as free radicals, increasing the burden of oxidative stress.

- Mimic chemical messengers in the body, causing disruption of biologic processes.

- Mimic hormones in the body—very likely a major contributing factor to breast and prostate cancers.

Toxins are detoxified in the liver in stages. In phase I, toxic compounds are neutralized. As previously discussed, this process generates a lot of free radicals. Neutralized toxins are then made water soluble for removal from the body during phase II (a process called conjugation). Conjugated-neutralized toxins are carried out of the liver in bile to be eliminated through the intestinal tract or are carried to the kidneys for removal. Diets heavy in processed food inhibit bile flow and cause retention of toxins. This accelerates any and all disease processes.

Most "normal" people seem to tolerate a certain level of toxins, but for recovery from CF/FMS, reducing the burden of toxins is essential. Xenobiotics can enter the body only by ingestion, inhalation, or absorption through skin. Avoiding processed food, incorporating organic foods, using only filtered water for beverages, and breathing clean air (indoors and out) can dramatically reduce the burden of toxins on the body. Many different herbal therapies offer liver protection and enhance the detoxification process.

SYSTEM DISRUPTOR #5: PHYSICAL STRESS

Three types of physical stress can affect your body: trauma, temperature, and pressure. Each one can be a significant factor in disease, and even everyday physical stress (minor trauma, being too cold or too hot, pressure changes) can aggravate CF/FMS symptoms and slow your recovery. For some people, extreme physical stress (severe trauma, severe hypothermia, severe hyperthermia, altitude sickness) can be the primary initiating factor setting the stage for CF/FMS to occur.

Physical stress certainly has the potential to be detrimental, but lack of any physical activity may be just as destructive. Common sense would suggest that being a couch potato would spare your bones, joints, and ligaments, but the opposite is actually true: Movement stimulates the healing systems of the body. Exercise generates endorphins, the pain-fighting "feel-good" chemicals that reduce pain and enhance repair functions. In fact, endorphins are an important key to your recovery. Regular exercise improves blood flow and helps remove toxins from your body. Continual movement is essential for life.

The direct downside of movement is friction. The friction caused by bones, joints, ligaments, and muscles coming in contact during movement is like rubbing two sticks together to create fire: Heat is produced and damage occurs. The body is well equipped to handle the damage caused by everyday movement, but if the healing systems of the body are compromised or if movement is excessive, inflammation results. Inflammation, as mentioned before, is the root cause of pain that occurs with CF/FMS.

A notch up from friction, trauma is a fact of life. Try getting through a day without minor bumps, scrapes, and bruises of some sort; it just isn't going to happen. Every time you bump, scrape, or bruise something, the healing mechanisms of your body immediately set about to repair the damage. Even when more significant trauma occurs, say falling off a ladder, a bruise or sore limb may be evident the next day but is usually gone within a week. Only when trauma becomes catastrophic does the body need outside help. Repair of lacerations, setting of broken bones, and sometimes surgery are required, but even these outside interventions are very dependent on the natural healing capacity of the body.

Beyond the stress of movement, extremes in temperature can be quite debilitating. If you are like most CF/FMS patients, you tend to feel cold in an environment where everyone else feels normal. People with CF/FMS generally feel most comfortable at a temperature range of 76–83 degrees. Although being warm enough is desirable, extreme heat can also be quite debilitating. Caution is advised when outside temperatures creep over 85 degrees, especially if physical activity is involved. Strenuous activity in temperatures greater than 90 degrees can set your recovery back for weeks, particularly if humidity is high.

The least obvious physical stress is pressure. All living things on the planet live at a fairly constant pressure defined by gravity and the surrounding atmosphere. We are all very dependent on this pressure—a fact well demonstrated by muscle wasting and loss of bone mass that occurs in astronauts in space. At the surface of the planet, however, only minor variations occur, primarily due to changes in weather. You may, like many people with CF/FMS, be very sensitive to these variations; low pressure systems are commonly associated with fatigue and aggravation of symptoms. Pressure can also be varied by altitude above and below sea level. Anyone can get altitude sickness above 8000 feet, but people with CF/FMS are much more susceptible.

For CF/FMS patients, there is a fine line between moving enough to gain benefit and crossing the line to a destructive process. Though regular exercise is a great idea, excessive exercise can slow your recovery. Pushing through won't do; excessive or intense exercise will just set you back. There must be a balance, exercising enough to generate endorphins and enhance blood flow, but not so much as to increase inflammation and compromise removal of toxins. This is a place where natural supplements can really help—omega-3 fatty acids (fish oil supplements) and herbal supplements reduce inflammation and promote optimal blood flow.

SYSTEM DISRUPTOR #6: ENERGY

Everything in the physical universe is made from energy, including the human body; like everyone else on the planet, you are a being of energy, and all the other energy sources in the universe have the potential to positively or negatively influence your energy. In fact, right now, your body is being bathed in a sea of energy. If you happen to be standing outside in bright sunshine or by a microwave transmission tower, the energy radiating toward your body is even more intense. Though living things have always had to deal with a certain amount of background radiation, the modern world has artificially increased exposure by an exponential amount. Different forms of energy affect living tissues in different ways.

Across the electromagnetic spectrum, radiation of energy can be defined as either ionizing or nonionizing. Ionizing radiation, which includes x-rays, gamma rays, and UV rays, acts very much like free radicals. Particles of energy pass through tissues and strike molecules, such as structural proteins and DNA, causing damage. At the other end of the spectrum, visible light, infrared, microwave, and radio waves are considered nonionizing because the energy produced does not directly damage tissue, but nonetheless, evidence is beginning to show that even these energetic particles can adversely affect human health.

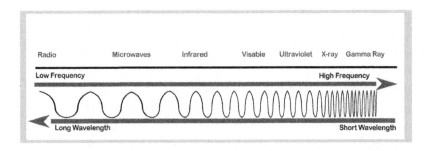

You and all other living things are exposed to a certain level of background radiation from gamma rays, x-ray and UV radiation from the earth, the sun, and space. Though these forms of radiation are a force of disease and aging, exposure from natural sources has been relatively constant since humans began walking the earth. Of more concern are the increased levels of radiation from artificial and unnatural sources. The following list provides a sampling of unnatural sources of radiation that could affect risk of disease.

- Over the past fifty years, there have been more than 2000 nuclear detonations for testing purposes and more than fifty accidents at nuclear plants. No one really knows how much this is affecting life-forms across the planet.

- Most everyone living in a developed country receives at least one x-ray procedure during a lifetime, and most people receive many. Though it is considered an acceptable risk and damage is minimal for most procedures, it is damage just the same. Ironically, the least healthy individuals are the most likely to undergo multiple diagnostic procedures and be exposed to the procedures with the highest concentration of x-rays.

- One silent source that can directly cause chronic fatigue (and increased risk of lung cancer) is radon gas. Radon is a decay product of uranium naturally present in soil. Because it exists as a very dense gas, it can collect underneath houses. In high-risk areas, collection of radon gas dramatically increases background radiation exposure to individuals living in the house. Fortunately, radon gas can be easily identified with a simple testing kit, and if it is present, shielding can be placed to minimize the risk.

- Any energy source, if intense enough, can produce heat and can damage living tissues. This is especially true of infrared and microwave radiation.[5]

---

[5] A 2011 study in Brazil (Dode et al., Science of the Total Environment) showed that people living within 500 meters of a cellular phone tower (microwave transmission) were 85% more likely to get cancer. The researchers looked at different towers around the country with different population groups and found the same result everywhere.

- Cellular phones may have been cleared of causing brain tumors (for the time being, anyway), but no one knows how much they affect brain function.

- CF/FMS sufferers often complain of feeling "out of sorts" after sitting by computers for a period of time. Not surprising, the human body is made of energy and radiates energy outwardly. The concern that human energy fields could be distorted or negatively affected by artificially generated energy is very real.

Quantitating the total contribution of artificial radiation to chronic disease and CF/FMS is challenging, but artifical radiation is a factor. If all artificial radiation were suddenly eliminated, the rate of chronic disease would probably drop significantly. Such an event is impossible, of course, but you can protect yourself from this silent threat. Antioxidants found in food and herbs offer protection against ionizing radiation. Many natural supplements have been defined (in both human and animal studies) to offer protection against ionizing radiation from radioactive sources. Electronic devices are now a permanent part of the modern world, but you can learn to live with them without being harmed.

System disruptors collectively set the stage for chronic infections with specific types of microbes. You (and everyone you come in contact with) are almost continually exposed to potentially pathogenic microbes. Most of these microbes, fortunately, have low potential to cause disease and pass by hardly noticed, but hardly noticed does not mean without potential for harm. If immune function is compromised, chronic low-grade infection can occur. These microbes are very stealthy—both difficult to diagnose and hard to eradicate. Once established, they hide inside cells and scavenge resources from the body. They have very sophisticated mechanisms of bypassing and compromising immune function. And unlike with more deadly microbes, killing you is not their goal; they want you alive for the valuable resources you provide...chronic means for a lifetime.

CHAPTER 3

THE ULTIMATE OPPORTUNISTS

M icrobes rule the world. They always have, and they always will. They outnumber us and outgun us, and they will still be here long after we are gone. Historically, infectious diseases (classic communicable diseases such as the plague, smallpox, cholera, malaria, and TB) have caused more death and destruction over the years than war and all other diseases combined. Infectious diseases are still a leading cause of death in the third world. In developed countries, modern antibiotics and vaccines have dramatically reduced the threat of the classical communicable diseases, but the spectrum of potentially pathogenic microbes is broad; microbes still play a major role in virtually all disease processes...including CF/FMS.

From a disease point of view, microbes can be loosely divided into two broad groups: normal flora and pathogens. They cannot be defined in terms of bad or good; they simply need resources for propagation. How they get those essential resources is what matters. Normal flora, the "friendly bacteria" that inhabit your gut and skin, have developed a symbiotic relationship with you; they get what they need without causing harm. In many cases, they actually provide benefit by inhibiting growth of other potential pathogens or breaking down substances in the gut to provide essential nutrients.

Pathogens are disease-causing microbes. Under the right circumstances, even normal flora can cross the line and become pathogens. E. coli (a normal gut flora) commonly causes urinary tract infections and can become a toxin-producing gut pathogen. An open wound is an invitation for a staph infection.

Virulence defines the ability of a pathogen to infect and cause disease. The most virulent pathogens take an aggressive breakdown-the-door approach, acquiring the resources they need and causing significant harm in the process. They are uninvited and must get through the barriers of the immune system to get what they want. Virulent pathogens are readily identified by the diseases they cause (strep throat, pneumonia, malaria, polio, smallpox, yellow fever, influenza, AIDS, etc.). They can be lethal, but their virulence is often their Achilles' heel. Because they are so visible, modern science has had significant success in defining them and creating tools that work against them—modern sanitation, antibiotics, and vaccines have dramatically reduced the threat of the most virulent microbes. High-virulence microbes are not the ones we worry about with CF/FMS.

Just possibly the most successful microbes are not the most virulent. Success in the microbe world is defined by the ability to propagate and flourish. Killing or severely disabling the host can be counterproductive. A stealthy approach offers great advantage. Persistence instead of virulence is how they win. Collectively, these microbes can be referred to as low-virulence pathogens.

Most everyone on the planet is frequently exposed to low-virulence pathogens, almost daily. Many of those pathogens never gain access beyond the initial barriers of the immune system and are hardly noticed. Some, however, do get a foot in the door, and a tug-of-war ensues between the microbe and the immune system until the offender is disposed of properly. If the immune system is compromised from the start or the microbe is stealthy enough, the gateway is left open for chronic infection to occur. Considering that much of the population lives in a state of immune compromise, associating pathogens of low virulence to chronic disease (and certainly CF/FMS) is not a challenge.

During an acute infection with one of these pathogens, the degree and nature of symptoms depend on the type of microbe, the site of initial infection, and the reaction of the immune system to the microbe or microbes (multi-microbial infections are not only possible but common—low-virulence pathogens tend to work together).

Mycoplasma pneumoniae, a very stealthy bacterium, provides a good example of a low-virulence pathogen—it is a common player in CF/FMS.

Infection with mycoplasma typically causes pharyngitis (sore throat), cough, fever, headache, malaise, rhinitis (runny nose), and eventually bronchitis and/or pneumonia (about the same symptoms as a bad cold or flu). After the initial tug-of-war (in the case of mycoplasma, about 3 weeks), the immune system gains ground and the host starts to recover. Subsequently, one of several things can occur:

- **The microbe is completely eradicated from the body— the host gets over it and eventually becomes completely well.** This is the most common scenario with any low-virulence microbe. How quickly it happens depends on the health of the immune system and whether secondary infections with other microbes has occurred (infection with one microbe often opens the door for other microbes to follow). Certain types of microbes (cold and flu viruses are good examples) can change antigenic presentation over time and can come back and infect the same person again, but at a separate event.

- **The microbe is suppressed such that it is no longer active but can become reactivated at a later time.** This is common with herpes viruses, which are harbored in nerve tissue and can reactivate if immune function is depressed. There are eight known herpes viruses that can infect humans, including herpes simplex 1 and 2, Varicella zoster (chickenpox—shingles), HH6, cytomegalovirus (CMV), and Epstein-Barr virus. Reactivation of herpes viruses is a common component of CF/FMS.

- **The microbe becomes an ill-fitting symbiotic organism that drains energy and resources from the body, but equilibrium occurs with the immune system such that the host remains without significant symptoms.** This may happen with many low-virulence microbes and may well be an under-recognized cause of progressive aging, chronic disease, and even cancer—you could be carrying something for years and not know it.

- **The microbe retains the upper hand and exists as an imbalanced symbiotic organism and remains in tug-of-war with the immune system, continuing to cause systemic symptoms that are seemingly unrelated to the initial infection.** This scenario occurs most often when the host's immune system is compromised. This is what happens with CF/FMS, Lyme disease, and possibly most autoimmune diseases.

Mycoplasma pneumoniae is a good example of a microbe that can fit into the latter two scenarios. If the bacterium is able to get past the initial site of infection (typically lungs with M. pneumoniae) and the barriers of the immune system, chronic systemic infection can occur. Symptoms associated with systemic infection are very different from the initial symptoms, which resolve completely over time. In other words, after the cough and congestion resolve, other seemingly unrelated symptoms such as fatigue and arthritis persist.

Mycoplasma are extremely small and, unlike most bacteria, do not have cell walls; therefore, they can take on different shapes and slip through spaces between cells. They can exist on the surface of cells but also readily grow inside cells, thus gaining protection from the immune system and antibiotic therapy...a really stealthy microbe.

Half the mycoplasma genome (genetic makeup) is devoted to manipulating the host's immune system. Mycoplasma routinely infect white blood cells and, at the same time, inhibit the ability of the white blood cell to properly dispose of the mycoplasma bacteria inside. They also block the ability of the immune system to recognize the infected cell as abnormal. (Normally, cells infected with viruses or bacteria are quickly targeted and destroyed.) In this manner, they can actually use the white blood cells to travel to sites of inflammation in the body (such as an inflamed joint).

Once on site, mycoplasma are able to induce inflammation by manipulating the signaling mechanisms of the immune system. Inflammation breaks down tissues and allows the bacteria to access the host's resources. Mitochondria are prime targets for energy; fatigue is always a factor in systemic mycoplasma infections. All tissues in the body can be infected with mycoplasma, but joints, muscles, and nerve tissue are favorite sites to scavenge resources. This results in arthritis, pain, fatigue, and neurological symptoms.

M. pneumoniae is not the only mycoplasma. There are more than 200 species of mycoplasma, and 23 are known to cause human illness. Some other types of mycoplasma enter the body via the intestinal tract and have a preference for infecting and destroying the villi of intestinal cells. A link between mycoplasma infection and food sensitivities would not be surprising. Villi are essential for absorption of nutrients, and chronic fatigue associated with weight loss and failure to thrive may be related to intestinal mycoplasma infection. Mycoplasma species with a preference for the genital tract have been associated with infertility and premature labor. These types of mycoplasma gain access by adhering to sperm.

Mycoplasma has been linked to both rheumatoid arthritis and multiple sclerosis. Very likely, it is a common player in CF/FMS (often in association with other microbes). Mycoplasma is known to facilitate the entry of viruses, such as HIV into cells (but likely it helps other viruses also). The way mycoplasma manipulate the immune system may have links to cancer (four different species of mycoplasma have been found inside different types of cancer cells). Transmission can occur through the respiratory tract, ingestion, sex, open wounds, and insect bites (ticks, biting flies, mosquitoes, fleas). Different species of mycoplasma may have a preferential route of infection, but they are all capable of any transmission route if the opportunity arises. Mycoplasma infection is extremely difficult to diagnose; the bacteria are very small, live inside cells, and change their antigenic presentation almost continually. The best protection from chronic mycoplasma infection is a healthy immune system.

Mycoplasma is just one microbe that has been associated with chronic fatigue. Borrelia burgdorferi, the primary microbe found in Lyme disease, could have been chosen as an example just as well. And there is not just one borrelia; at least two other species of borrelia (that we know of) can cause Lyme disease. Borrelia is the most sinister of all the stealth bacteria, and Lyme disease is possibly the most underdiagnosed, inappropriately treated, and misunderstood disease of our time. The number of people diagnosed with CF/FMS who are infected with borrelia is unknown.

Borrelia is a spirochete. Spirochetes are shaped like corkscrews and have the unique ability to bore deeply into collagenous tissue. Collagen is a nutrient source, and high-collagen areas including joints, skin, brain, and heart are favorite sites of invasion. Borrelia also has the ability to shed the spirochete armor and thrive inside cells (like other pathogens common to CF/FMS), shielding it from the immune system and antibiotics. Borrelia has extraordinarily sophisticated mechanisms of inhibiting and outsmarting the immune system. It changes its antigenic presentation continually. This, and the fact that blood levels are very low make Borrelia difficult to diagnose and even more difficult to get rid of. Borrelia infections can be accompanied by other tick-borne pathogens, including bartonella, babesia, ehrlichia, mycoplasma, and possibly others still unknown. Multiple pathogens always complicate the picture even further.

The range of pathogenic bacteria found in CF/FMS patients is certainly not limited to tick bites. Different species of mycoplasma can be acquired from airborne particles, ingestion, and sexual contact in addition to tick bites. In studies where chronic fatigue syndrome patients are tested for bacterial diseases, mycoplasma stands out as the most common offender, but other bacteria have also been found. Chlamydia pneumoniae (causes pneumonia initially) and Brucella species (acquired from unpasteurized milk products) have also been implicated in fatigue syndromes. And these are just a few that have been identified; who knows how many are yet to be recognized.

An interesting trait that all of these bacteria have in common is the ability to live inside cells. Adapting to intracellular existence protects the bacteria from the immune system and antibiotics. When it comes to true microbial success, microbes that thrive inside cells are the champions...and they are much more common than most people recognize.

Chronic fatigue patients often complain of having a flu that never goes away. Flu-like symptoms are common with viral infections, and reactivations of viral infections are not unusual in CF/FMS. The three most common are Epstein-Barr virus (EBV), the cause of mononucleosis; Cytomegalovirus (CMV), a common viral infection that can cause heart failure; and human herpesvirus type 6 (HHV-6), a virus very commonly found active in chronic fatigue patients. All three are herpes-type viruses. As mentioned previously, eight known herpes-type viruses can infect humans. The list includes herpes simplex type 1 (fever blisters), herpes simplex type 2 (genital ulcers), and varicella-zoster virus (chickenpox and shingles). A common feature all of these viruses share is the ability to lie dormant in nerve tissue and reemerge later when immune system function is compromised. Chronic viral infections causing fatigue are not limited to herpes viruses. Hepatitis B and C can remain as low-grade infections of the liver for a lifetime.

Fungi also play a role in CF/FMS, but not in the same way as bacteria and viruses. Infections with true pathogenic fungal species are extremely debilitating and relatively rare; they are not typical players in CF/FMS. More commonly, chronic exposure to toxic mold spores (present in an enclosed damp environment, such as an old house) induces immune compromise that allows low-virulence microbes already present to flourish. Eradicating any sources of mold spores in your living space is essential for overcoming CF/FMS.

The only fungal "infection" commonly associated with CF/FMS is Candida species. Candida is a benign yeast that exists ubiquitously everywhere. Candida is present on your skin and inside your gut. It only becomes a problem under just the right circumstances. An imbalance in vaginal flora can result in a vaginal yeast infection, and imbalances in gut flora can allow overgrowth. Candida is an opportunist that thrives in immune-compromised hosts. Candida loves sugar; avoiding sugar and simple starches is essential for overcoming CF/FMS. Candida, however, is not aggressive enough to be considered a direct cause of CF/FMS; it's simply part of the problem. Generally, it will resolve spontaneously as measures are taken to improve immune function, but specific treatment can enhance recovery if candida is specifically diagnosed.

Protozoa (a life-form slightly higher on the evolutionary scale than bacteria) can cause fatigue and can become chronic but are less commonly associated with CF/FMS. Pathogenic protozoa typically cause specific symptoms that define the disease process. The best example is malaria characterized by relapsing fevers and anemia. The protozoa that causes malaria is spread by mosquitos and infects red blood cells. Malaria is a high-virulence pathogen that commonly kills people. Babesia, a similar protozoan infection transmitted by ticks (sometimes associated with Lyme disease), also infects and destroys red blood cells, but infections are milder and often self-limited. In comparison to malaria, babesia rarely kills people and should be considered a low-virulence pathogen. Babesia can occasionally become part of the CF/FMS picture, but making a firm diagnosis is challenging.

All the pathogens typically associated with CF/FMS share similar qualities:

- They are low-virulence. Not everyone infected will develop a chronic infection or ever show symptoms (acutely or chronically).

- They are not considered major disease-causing pathogens by conventional medicine.

- Immune compromise seems to be a prerequisite for developing a chronic infection.

- Symptoms of chronic infection are very different than of acute infection; chronic infections typically cause chronic fatigue and related symptoms.

- Chronic infections with these microbes do not kill people directly (but they can make life miserable for a long time).

- These pathogens thrive inside cells, thus gaining protection from the immune system and antibiotics.

- These pathogens are experts at evading and compromising the immune system at key points.

- These pathogens are synergistic—infection with one pathogen makes it easier for infections with other low-virulence pathogens to occur.

The above qualities make such pathogens difficult to diagnose and even more difficult to eradicate once they become established. The ones discussed are just a sampling of the pathogens that we know something about; others yet unknown may well exist. Just because something isn't recognized doesn't mean it isn't there. Who knows how many undiscovered low-virulence pathogens are lurking about and possibly already play a role in CF/FMS!

In 1975, a "new" disease was discovered in Lyme, Connecticut, and within a couple of years, the causative microbe, Borrelia burgdorferi, was identified and named. Now defined as an emerging disease, Lyme disease is suddenly being diagnosed commonly all across the country. Seemingly unrelated, in 1991, the mummified remains of a human male (approximate age 45) were recovered from a melting glacier in the Alps of Europe. Very interestingly, this ancient human, locked in ice for 5,300 years, harbored the same bacteria as the one causing today's supposed new-age disease. Tissue samples from an autopsy done on those remains in 2010 revealed the characteristic genetic signature of Borrelia burgdorferi. But, of course, the man didn't die of Lyme disease; an arrow in the back piercing a major blood vessel was what did him in![6]

---

[6] "Iceman Autopsy," Stephen S. Hall, *National Geographic* magazine, November 2011.

Microbe Connections to CF/FMS

The possibility of hidden microbes being a primary underlying factor in chronic fatigue-type syndromes (and also autoimmune diseases[7]) is hard to ignore, but absolutely determining exactly which microbes are present is nearly impossible. Because the types of pathogenic microbes found in CF/FMS thrive inside cells and isolated locations in the body, finding them and eradicating them is a real challenge. A positive diagnosis of one microbe does not exclude the presence of other hidden microbes (possibly even some yet to be identified by modern science), and they all work synergistically. (Microbes have been successfully playing this game for a lot longer than we have!)

The microbes involved in CF/FMS have evolved intricate mechanisms of disabling or tricking key parts of the immune system. Some of these mechanisms have been defined, but much is still unknown. Each different pathogen has evolved different mechanisms of disrupting immune function. What happens to the immune system when a host is infected with multiple low-virulence pathogens simultaneously is a huge question that still remains. Likely, this happens more often than not, and it may explain variations in symptoms and also variations in immune dysfunction.

No two patients with CF/FMS are exactly alike. Differences are caused by variation in exposure to system disruptors, the patient's genetic makeup, and the types of pathogens present. Compromise of immune function is a common denominator in every case, but types of immune dysfunction can vary. Certain patients present with muscle pain and no joint pain, or no pain at all; these cases may be predominantly viral. Viruses are also more apt to directly affect the liver. Joint inflammation and migrating arthritis may indicate predominant bacterial involvement; borrelia (Lyme disease) and mycoplasma are common culprits (but others are possible). Intestinal mycoplasma may be a factor in patients with severe food sensitivities, weight loss, and failure to thrive. Some of the sickest

---

[7] See Appendix A for a primer on how the immune system works and a possible explanation of why these diseases sometimes progress to autoimmune disease.

chronic fatigue patients display immune suppression across the board. These patients' situations have been given the designation Chronic Fatigue Immune Dysfunction Syndrome (CFIDS); very likely, multiple microbes are involved.

Where We Go from Here

The old target-and-destroy approach just doesn't apply. Conventional medications have value but are limited in scope. Drugs can reduce symptoms and offer acute benefit, but overuse can actually inhibit recovery. Antibiotics are indicated for acute infections but have less value when infection with an intracellular pathogen becomes chronic, when there are multiple pathogens, or when there are unidentified pathogens (in other words, most of the time). Systemic steroid therapy is sometimes necessary to suppress destructive immune overactivity, but steroids do not restore normal immune function or eradicate infections (in fact, systemic steroids may prolong infections).

Restoration of normal immune function is the only way to overcome CF/FMS. Reducing system disruptors contributing to immune dysfunction is the first order of business. This is the part where you, the patient, must take an active role; only you can save yourself. The restoration process can be enhanced with natural therapies. Supplemental antioxidants reduce damage to cells and tissues. Adaptogenic herbs balance hormones, increase stress resistance, and restore balance to the immune system. Herbs providing broad-spectrum antimicrobial properties are extremely important for overcoming CF/FMS. In fact, restoration of normal health is unlikely without embracing natural therapies. (Plants have also been successfully playing this game for a very long time—again, much longer than we have!)

You have now reached a crossroad. You are clinging to the stone walls inside a cold dark well called chronic fatigue, but you now have the information that can get you out. Choices. You can stay where you are, palliating symptoms with drugs or other therapies but not moving up or down…or…you can gather all your resources and make the climb out! The climb out is not as difficult as it might seem. Right now, your ability to climb is being hindered by superficial attachments that are holding you down. The next chapter will help you define those attachments and measure the state of your present health.

CHAPTER 4

ESTABLISHING A BASELINE

Before going anywhere, you have to know where you are. Knowing your present state of health will help you define progress. Though you may know intuitively how bad or good your health is right now, it is useful to quantitate that information. The following questionnaire, self-exam, and list of labs will help you establish a baseline.

HEALTH PRACTICES

Complete the following questionnaire (honestly, please). The answers should reflect the past couple of years of your life, not the past several weeks. Notice that each question is set up a little bit differently. Write down the number beside your choice on a separate sheet of paper and add up all the numbers at the end. Don't get too uptight about specifics; we're looking for general trends here.

DIETARY HISTORY

Grain-fed meat (pork, beef) consumption:
(0) frequently/daily   (1) 1–2 x weekly   (2) never/1–2 x monthly

Processed meat (sausage, hot dogs) consumption:
(0) frequently/daily   (1) 1–2 x weekly   (2) never/1–2 x monthly

Dairy (milk, cheese) consumption:
(0) frequently/daily   (1) 1–2 x weekly   (2) never/1–2 x monthly

Poultry consumption:
(0) frequently/daily   (1) never/rarely   (2) 1–2 x weekly

Fish/Seafood consumption:
(0) never/rarely   (1) occasionally   (2) often (1–3 x weekly)

Free-range local farm eggs:
(0) never/rarely   (1) occasionally   (2) often (2–4 x weekly)

Servings of fresh vegetables daily:
(0) 0–1   (1) 2–4   (3) ≥5

Servings of fresh fruit daily:
(0) 0–1   (1) ≥5   (2) 2–4

Bean (any type) consumption:
(0) never/rarely   (1) occasionally   (2) frequently/daily

Cruciferous vegetable (e.g., broccoli, cabbage) consumption:
(0) never/rarely   (1) occasionally   (2) frequently

Yogurt consumption:
(0) never/rarely   (1) occasionally   (2) frequently/daily

Nut (other than peanuts) consumption:
(0) never/rarely   (1) occasionally   (2) frequently/daily

Percentage of food wrapped or packaged (processed food):
(0) >70%   (1) 30–70%   (3) <30%

Cake, cookies, pastry consumption:
(0) frequently/daily   (1) 1–2 x weekly   (2) never/1–2 x monthly

Bread and other products made with flour:
(0) frequently/daily   (1) 1–2 x weekly   (2) never/1–2 x
monthly

HEALTH HISTORY
Exercise:
(0) never/rarely   (1) occasionally   (3) frequently/daily

Practice relaxation or breathing exercises:
(0) never/rarely   (1) occasionally   (3) frequently/daily

Average hours of sleep per night:
(0) <4   (1) 4–6   (3) ≥ 7

Cigarette smoking:
(0) still smoking   (2) quit for >1 year   (3) never

Alcohol consumption:
(0) >2 drinks/day   (1) 1–2 drinks/day   (2) 3 or less/week

Tolerate stress:
(0) poorly   (1) okay   (3) well

Have teeth cleaned
(0) never/rarely   (1) once or less/year   (2) twice/year

Drink filtered water or liquids that have been filtered:
(0) rarely   (1) occasionally   (2) most of the time

Work:
(0) work overtime frequently or disabled   (2) work a normal
30–40 hours

I enjoy my work (stay-at-home moms qualify):
(0) rarely   (1) occasionally   (2) most of the time

My work requires travel:
(0) often   (1) occasionally   (2) rarely

A musty smell is present in my home and/or workplace:
(0) most of the time   (1) not very strong   (2) not present

Add up your score. A perfect score is 67. Of course, the worst score is 0. Most people score somewhere in the middle. Your goal, of course, is improvement. You may have recognized that all the favorable answers are on the right and the less desirable answers are on the left. This will help guide you in areas that need the most effort. Repeat the questionnaire after several months to see if you have a better score. Generally, a better score parallels feeling better.

SELF-EXAM

A great deal of useful information can be determined from self-analysis. This is not the same as self-diagnosis; it is simply an exercise in self-awareness. The information gathered can guide health practices toward restoring normal in the body. It can also be useful information to pass along to your healthcare provider (most of them do not have time anymore to ask these basic important questions).

Stool analysis. Stools are a taboo topic in daily conversation, but stools can provide a wealth of information about the digestive tract.

> **Frequency.** Normal bowel movements consist of soft but formed stools that occur spontaneously 1–2 times daily. Gas and bloating are minimal.

- Constipation is defined as the absence of spontaneous bowel movements. Stools are generally hard. Flatulence is common. Frequency is generally less than once daily. Constipation occurs as a result of impaired colonic activity caused by over-consumption of processed food. Excessive laxative use can damage the colon and impair motility. Some individuals are more prone to constipation than others.

- Loose stools in the form of poorly formed or liquid stools, typically occurring more than once daily, are a sign of impaired digestion and gut inflammation. When accompanied by gas and bloating (usually present), loose stools are a sign of abnormal bacterial overgrowth.

Undigested food. Nuts, such as sunflower seeds and pumpkin seeds, and corn typically come through undigested, but other food substances should not be identifiable. Loose stools containing undigested food are a strong sign of low acid production in the stomach and low digestive enzymes. In this case, digestive enzyme supplements and vinegar (2 tbsp. apple cider vinegar in 6 oz. water) with meals can be very beneficial.

Color. The normal color of stool is reddish-brown. The color represents bile in stool, which is necessary for digesting fat. Light-grey stools suggest stagnant bile production from the liver and gallbladder. Tar-like stools can represent bleeding in the stomach, and significant amounts of bright red blood are never a good sign.

Float or not. Normal stools sink. Floating stools, especially if loose and light grey, indicate poor digestion of fat. It is a sign of insufficient enzyme production from the pancreas and stagnant bile production.

Odor. Normal stools have odor, but odor strong enough to run you out of the bathroom is a strong sign of extreme bacterial imbalance. Foul-smelling flatulence is just as indicative.

Urine. Adequate urine flow indicates normal hydration. If you are drinking the right amount, urine will be the color of lemonade. Normal voiding should occur several times daily and 1–2 times at night. If your urine is as clear as water, you are probably over-hydrating. Urine the color of apple juice indicates dehydration. Urine should not have a foul odor (unless asparagus has been consumed).

Everyone always wants to know exactly how much to drink, but the answer is very dependent on physical activity and sweating. Color of urine is the best guide. Don't forget: Vegetables and fruit contain high quantities of water compared to processed food, which generally contains little moisture.

Blood glucose. Abnormally elevated insulin levels and elevated blood glucose levels are major system disruptors. Self-monitoring with a glucometer obtained from a pharmacy is a good practice in self-awareness of carbohydrate consumption. The finger-sticks are not that bad when you get used to them. Use an automatic lance and stick on the side of your finger instead of on the pad, where the nerves are. Measure fasting blood glucose in the morning before eating and post-prandial (after eating) blood glucose two hours after a main meal. Your target is blood glucose <90 mg/dl fasting and <110 mg/dl postprandial.

Tongue. The Chinese have been studying tongues for thousands of years, and whole encyclopedias are devoted to diagnosing disease by tongue analysis. The tongue is a barometer for the rest of the body. Although in-depth analysis is rarely indicated, an examination in the mirror can provide valuable information.

The surface of a normal tongue is wet, pink, and mildly grooved. Dryness with white or yellow plaque across the surface and associated burning is a sign of poor digestion, immune compromise, and intestinal bacterial imbalance. It can also represent a yeast infection (thrush). Improvement in tongue health generally follows improved health in general, but thrush must be diagnosed and treated by a healthcare provider.

Back of Throat. The back of the throat is actually a great barometer for airborne toxins. A scratchy throat in the absence of a viral infection often indicates the presence of threatening toxins in the environment and a debilitated state of health. As your health improves, you will become less sensitive to toxic threats.

Pulse. Average pulse is 72 beats/minute. Find your pulse by palpating the outer portion of the opposite upturned wrist, just on the other side of the largest tendon. Check for consistency; beats should occur very regularly. Count each pulse for 30 seconds, and multiply by two.

- Consistent low pulse rate (<60) can be an indication of hypothyroidism, compromised immune status, and/or compromised adrenal function.

- Low pulse rate associated with exercise intolerance, and persistent low rate with exercise can be a sign of heart block (can occur in Lyme disease); this needs direct attention by a doctor.

- Irregular pulse with skipped beats can be sign of microbial infection of the heart, especially if accompanied by chest pain (heart involvement is somewhat common in Lyme disease) and also needs attention from a doctor.

- Persistent elevated pulse during rest (>100) should also be brought to the attention of your healthcare provider.

Body temperature. Average temperature is 98.6°F, but variations are normal. Temperature is generally lowest first thing in the morning and higher during the day. Exercise can raise body temperature. Temperature varies during different times in the menstrual cycle and increases with pregnancy. Basal body temperature (BBT) is taken by oral thermometer (digital preferred) first thing in the morning, before your feet hit the floor. Consistent BBT <97.5° is a possible indication of low metabolism, which could indicate hypothyroidism. High temperature (>99°) could indicate an active infection.

Pain. Pain is very commonly associated with chronic fatigue and is a hallmark feature of fibromyalgia. Pain is generally associated with inflammation and is generally limited to the area of body that is inflamed, but this is not always the case; pain can be referred. Pain associated with other symptoms (fever and vomiting, for example) is generally more concerning than isolated pain. Any unexplained pain, severe pain, worsening pain, or pain associated with other symptoms should immediately be brought to the attention of a healthcare provider. Resolution of pain is one of the most positive (and desirable) indications of getting well.

LABORATORY TESTING

There is, of course, no test that specifically diagnoses chronic fatigue or fibromyalgia. In conventional medical terms, chronic fatigue and fibromyalgia are diagnoses of exclusion. When nothing else fits, it might be CF/FMS. There is value, however, in quantifying general health information. Also, laboratory testing can uncover hidden disease processes—fatigue is associated with most chronic diseases.

The following list is meant as a very general guide. It is very important to ask how much a test will influence your therapy before ordering that test—some commonly ordered tests actually have limited value in defining therapy. Your healthcare provider can help you choose specific labs offering the highest probability of benefit and also can help you interpret those tests. Ranges of normal vary from lab to lab, and your healthcare provider can help you define a truly abnormal test.

Please note that none of the lab tests discussed below is an absolute prerequisite for following the advice provided in this book; they are provided for informational purposes to help you understand tests that your healthcare provider may order.

General Testing

General Blood Chemistries

- **Electrolytes**. Sodium, potassium, chloride, and CO_2 are generally normal, unless you are really sick.

- **RBC Magnesium**. Low magnesium is sometimes a factor in CF/FMS

- **Liver function**. Abnormal values suggest an elevated rate of liver compromise, possibly from toxins or viruses such as hepatitis. Elevated bilirubin suggests increased breakdown and turnover of red blood cells. Certain low-virulence microbes (bartonella, for example) destroy red blood cells.

- **Kidney function**. BUN and creatinine screen for kidney disease.

- **Lipid studies**. Cholesterol commonly increases with age. Elevated cholesterol is associated with decline in liver function that occurs with age. The nutrition guidelines in this book are actually very good for lowering cholesterol. Significantly elevated cholesterol, however, should be addressed by your healthcare provider.

Urinalysis

- **pH**. Urine pH should be consistently alkaline, reflecting high consumption of vegetables and fruit.

- **WBCs, nitrites**. These tests show evidence of urinary tract infection.

- **Protein**. Elevated levels can indicate kidney disease.

- **Bilirubin**. Elevated levels show increased turnover of red blood cells.

Complete Blood Count with Differential (CBC with Diff)

- **White blood cell count (WBC)**. Low WBC (<4000) can indicate chronic infection with virus or low-virulence bacteria, but also commonly occurs in normal people. Elevated WBC (>11,500) can be an indication of active infection.

- **Hemoglobin (Hb)**. Anemia is indicated by Hb <12.0. Anemia can be caused by blood loss (heavy periods), inadequate production of RBCs (chemotherapy), and increased destruction of RBCs (infection—malaria is a prime example, but there are others). Hb levels >16.0 can be associated with smoking, living at altitude, and having excessive iron stores in the body.

Markers for Oxidative Stress

C-reactive protein (CRP). CRP is possibly the best marker presently available for measuring inflammation (oxidative stress). It is also a good marker for general health status; high levels (>10) correlate with increased risk of disease. Normal levels, however, are often seen in CF/FMS patients who follow relatively good dietary habits. Even without clinical markers, however, the benefit from consuming high concentrations of antioxidants from food and natural supplements is highly beneficial.

Metabolic Testing

Glucose Metabolism

Excessive carbohydrate consumption is a major system disrupter that must be controlled before overcoming CF/FMS. Three primary tests—fasting blood glucose, hemoglobin A1c, and fasting insulin—define insulin resistance and abnormal glucose metabolism.

- **Fasting blood glucose**. Levels >100 mg/dl suggest pre-diabetes. Levels >126 mg/dl suggest overt diabetes.

- **Fasting insulin**. Levels defined as elevated suggest insulin resistance (normal range varies depending on the lab). Insulin resistance is a factor contributing to immune dysfunction and hormone imbalances.

- **Hemoglobin A1c (HbA1c)**. HbA1c measures the cumulative damage done by excessive carbohydrate consumption. Ideal is 4.8%–5.2%. Levels >5.6% indicate pre-diabetes. Levels >6.4% indicate overt diabetes.

Thyroid Function

Complete thyroid function should include thyroid stimulating hormone (TSH), free T_4, free T_3, and thyroid antibodies. Diseases associated with abnormal thyroid function and CF/FMS share many common symptoms, and the two are often found together. Correcting of abnormal thyroid function can accelerate recovery. Testing for thyroid antibodies (TPO and thyroglobulin) is important to identify Hashimoto's disease, a form of autoimmune thyroid dysfunction.

Vitamins

Any vitamins can be tested for, but the vitamin levels that offer the most value include vitamin D, vitamin B12, and RBC folate.

- **Vitamin B12**. Low B12 levels (normal ranges vary between labs) can be a sign of low intake (as in vegetarians) but are more commonly a sign of inadequate absorption and gastric dysfunction. Vitamin B12 generally increases spontaneously with improved health habits, but in the short term, B12 injections or sublingual (under the tongue) supplements can improve energy levels. Activated forms of B12 are better absorbed orally than the more common inactive forms used in most multivitamin products.

- **RBC folate**. Folate is important for many functions in the body. Many people take folic acid supplements, but 40% of the population metabolize folic acid poorly (folic acid is not a natural folate). Supplementing with natural folates (methyltetrahydrofolate or folinic acid) is preferred.

- **Vitamin D**. Vitamin D is not only important for healthy bones but also very important for normal immune function. There are several forms of vitamin D. Calcidiol (25(OH) D) is the most commonly measured form in blood tests. Normal ranges for blood levels of Vitamin D and indications for supplementation are both controversial. The Institute of Medicine officially defines calcidiol levels >20 ng/ml as normal and >50 ng/ml as too high. The Institute of Medicine's recommendations for daily vitamin D include sun exposure or 600–1000 IU of vitamin D3 daily. The Vitamin D Council, however, recommends 40–100 ng/ml as the normal range, generally requiring much higher doses of supplementation. Levels of >40 ng/ml have been associated with reduced risk of many cancers and chronic disease in general. Maintaining vitamin D levels >40 ng/ml is recommended for CF/FMS recovery. Have your levels checked every 3–6 months.

Hormone Testing

Adrenal

Adrenal dysfunction is a given in CF/FMS. Elevated cortisol levels, associated with increased physical and emotional stress, contribute to sleeplessness and other symptoms. Prolonged adrenal stress can result in decreased cortisol levels, with symptoms of extreme fatigue. Because adrenal dysfunction is always present in CF/FMS and generally normalizes with proper treatment, measurement of adrenal hormone levels is generally not necessary. On rare occasions when a patient is not improving, measurement of cortisol can be beneficial. The best measure is salivary cortisol, measured 4 times over 24 hours.

Reproductive

Menopause can exacerbate symptoms of CF/FMS. Though usually obvious, in the absence of periods, menopause can be confirmed by an elevated pituitary hormone called FSH. Levels >25 IU/ml indicate menopause. Other hormone levels, including estrogen and progesterone, are generally not necessary to measure, but measuring them may be recommended by your healthcare provider. In men with CF/FMS, testing of total and free testosterone is sometimes indicated.

Autoimmune Disease

The causative factors for CF/FMS and autoimmune diseases are the same, and it is not unusual for CF/FMS to progress to some type of autoimmune disease (a continuum of disease severity, rather than different diseases). Testing for autoimmune disease can be beneficial, though any chronic disease process often improves with the recovery protocol. Your healthcare provider can help you with specific testing if indicated.

- **Rheumatoid factor** should be a standard test if severe arthritis is present.
- **ANA titer** is positive in many types of autoimmune disease.

Immune Function

Many experts have tried to find a specific pattern for immune dysfunction for CF/FMS, but as of yet, one has not emerged. Though immune dysfunction is universally present in CF/FMS patients, patterns of immune dysfunction vary widely. This is probably because of the wide spectrum of possible microbes that can be involved.

Some providers test extensively for markers of immune dysfunction, but until specific patterns are defined, immune testing has limited value. One of the extraordinary benefits of natural herbal therapy is restoration of normal immune function, no matter the type of dysfunction present. This, in itself, obviates the need for expensive immune testing.

Microbes

Low-virulence pathogens (bacterial and viral are most common, but protozoan or fungal are also possible) are almost universally present in CF/FMS, autoimmune diseases, and many other chronic diseases; often, however, they are difficult to detect and define. Detection of a specific microbe can focus treatment but can also potentially be misleading if multiple low-virulence pathogens are present. In addition, low-virulence pathogens with potential to cause CF/FMS may exist that have not been identified. Testing is most important for a patient who is not getting well.

- **Lyme disease**. Borrelia is recognized as a common underlying factor in many cases of CF/FMS. Early recognition and treatment is important in all cases of tick bite.

  - The ELISA test, commonly used for screening, is actually not sensitive enough for screening and should not be used.

  - Western blot is presently the most accurate test but still has significant limitations. The occurrence of new strains of the causative bacterium have rendered twenty-year-old testing modalities to be of limited value; diagnosis is often left to a high index of suspicion.

  - **I-spot Lyme test**. This is a new test as of March 2013. It tests for immune cells (T-cells) with memory specific to Borrelia. The test is reported to be much more specific and sensitive than the Western blot but is awaiting FDA approval. The cost is $375–$400, presently not covered by insurance.

A positive test for Borrelia can guide therapy, but a negative test does not rule out the possibility of Borrelia being present, or the presence of other microbes.

- **Mycoplasma.** Testing is available for certain species of mycoplasma, including nasal swabs and blood testing for Mycoplasma pneumoniae and genital swabs for mycoplasma/Ureaplasma. The question is whether or not to test. Because testing has many false negatives and testing for many species of mycoplasma is not widely available, it's almost better to assume for the possibility of mycoplasma, unless there are specific indications for testing—such as persistent bronchitis/pneumonia or chronic pelvic infections.

- **Yeast/fungal infections.** Chronic yeast infections and other fungal infections are common in immune-compromised individuals, especially if high processed carbohydrate consumption is a factor. Dietary modifications, probiotics, and restoration of normal immune function and herbal therapy generally eradicate yeast. Occasionally, prescription antifungal medications are indicated. Testing is indicated only if chronic fatigue and gastrointestinal symptoms are not resolving with therapy.

  - Blood tests IgG, IgA, IgM antibodies for Candida—high titers indicate overgrowth.

  - Stool cultures for Candida overgrowth

  - Urine testing for Candida waste product called D-arabinitol (Urine Organix Dysbiosis Test)

- **Viral testing.** Viruses commonly associated with CFS include Epstein-Barr virus, CMV, and HHV-6. Most people are exposed to one or all of these viruses at an early age and the viruses lie dormant within tissues. Reactivation of these viruses is very common in CF/FMS; therefore, testing is rarely indicated.

- **Tuberculosis.** TB can be a cause of chronic fatigue. Chest x-ray and TB test are indicated if fevers and cough are present.

- **Hepatitis.** Hepatitis screen for B and C are indicated if risk factors are present or liver function is abnormal.

- **Sexually transmitted diseases**. Testing for HIV and/or syphilis may be indicated if exposure is a concern. Testing for gonorrhea, chlamydia, and genital mycoplasma is performed with a genital swab.

Toxins

- **Heavy metals**. Buildup of heavy metals and other toxins can be a hidden factor in CF/FMS. Every person living on the planet today is carrying some heavy metals, but no one really knows how much is enough to cause disease. The biggest source of concern is amalgam dental fillings. Talk to your healthcare provider. If heavy-metal toxicity is a concern, testing can be performed.

- **Organic toxins**. The presence of organic toxins (pesticides, plastic residues) is almost a given and can be addressed with dietary and lifestyle modifications.

- **Food sensitivities**. Chronic gastrointestinal dysfunction is often associated with sensitivities to commonly consumed foods (not the same as food allergies, such as peanut allergy). Symptoms associated with food sensitivities are commonly delayed for 1–2 days after the food is consumed. Typical symptoms include fatigue, joint pain, muscle pain, and general achiness—in fact, food sensitivities alone can be the root of CF/FMS.

Food sensitivities are best defined by an elimination diet—a diet designed to selectively identify and eliminate problem foods (a basic elimination diet is included in the "Purify" chapter). Problem foods can also be delineated with specific IgG testing. A basic food-sensitivity panel can be obtained for about $120. This shows general categories of foods to be avoided. Generally, food sensitivities resolve as health improves.

- **Comprehensive stool analysis**. Stool analysis is valuable for defining gastrointestinal dysfunction and for diagnosing parasites and yeast overgrowth. This expensive test is generally reserved for extreme cases, when dietary modifications and supplements are not enough to overcome gastrointestinal problems.

Miscellaneous

- **Omega-3/Omega-6 ratio**. The ratio of omega-3 fatty acids to omega-6 fatty acids is an important marker for balance of inflammatory factors in the body. Testing guides proper supplementation.

- **Ferritin**. Ferritin measures iron stores. Low iron stores or excessively high iron stores can be a contributing cause of chronic fatigue.

Knowing the state of your present health is important for getting better. Lab tests can be helpful in that regard, but testing should be limited to lab tests that you and your healthcare provider decide offer the highest probability of providing useful information. Now that you know where you stand, it's time to move on to supportive therapies that can make your life a whole lot better.

PART TWO

ESSENTIAL SUPPORT

The stone walls of the CF/FMS well are wet, cold, and slippery; it's easy to lose your grip. I was about to lose my grip forever when I found my lifeline in the form of natural herbal supplements. Natural herbal therapies are particularly beneficial for creating a healing environment within the body. Combinations of herbs, blended together for synergy, suppress hidden microbes, restore normal immune function, reduce inflammation, provide antioxidant protection, and balance hormones. In short, herbs restore normal. And they do it with very low potential for side effects and toxicity. Compared to virtually all other therapies, the herbs discussed in this section are forgiving, safe, and easy to use.

Drugs also have a place in treatment, but mostly for reducing symptoms and inhibiting the destructive processes of disease. Early on, this can be very important, but as healing occurs, the need for drug therapy declines.

Beyond conventional drug therapy and medical procedures, there are scores of alternative therapies, all of which offer potential benefit, but few of which are backed by good science. Even so, the risk associated with most alternative therapies is generally very low—they can play an important role in your recovery process.

CHAPTER 5

ENHANCE HEALING

The focus of this chapter is on enhancing the normal healing capacity of the body. The body has an extraordinary capacity for healing; you just need to know how to tap into it. Symptom reduction is important, but it should not come at the expense of restoring normal health. All of the therapies discussed in this chapter are designed to give you a jump start on the healing process.

Drug therapy for symptom control is a common starting point for many people; you may already be taking one or several pharmaceuticals. Very likely, however, you wouldn't mind getting off those drugs; side effects of some type are almost universally present. Be patient; you will reach a point where you will need them less and possibly not at all. Healing comes first, and healing takes time. It will happen. If you are habituated to a drug, it may take extra effort (preferably guided by a qualified healthcare provider), but it can happen just the same. Drugs can be slowly tapered as your health starts to rebound.

Of all drug therapies, antibiotics are possibly the most important in the healing process. If you have been specifically diagnosed with a microbial infection such as Lyme disease or mycoplasma, antibiotics may be indicated, especially if the infection is recent and acute. Once chronic infections with low-virulence microbes become established, however, conventional antibiotics become less valuable. Chronic low-virulence infections are often best managed with herbal therapies having antimicrobial properties. These types of herbs can be used long term at high doses without concerns of disrupting normal flora or of causing gastrointestinal side effects. Natural herbal therapies can be used along with conventional antibiotics.

Natural therapies are the absolute best way to tap into the remarkable healing potential of the human body. Natural supplements can be started immediately, and the only habit you have to learn is remembering to take the supplements a couple of times a day. The list of natural supplements provided in this book is a good place to start, but the list is not, by any means, exclusive. It is simply a logically derived collection of supplements that offer a high probability of providing benefit. Over time, you will probably gradually modify your daily regimen as you learn more about natural supplements. The references provided at the end of the book offer great resources for more extensive study of these and other natural supplements!

On your own, you may also want to explore other alternative therapies. There are many choices—massage therapy, Reiki and other forms of energy medicine, acupuncture, and more. Most have very low potential for harm and complement any of the recommendations made in this book. The biggest limitation of these therapies is cost.

NATURAL THERAPY OPTIONS

Many natural therapies offer benefit for chronic fatigue recovery. The list I provide has been consolidated down to a reasonable assortment of suggestions offering the highest potential for benefit with the lowest potential for toxicity. Many natural therapies provide more than one benefit. In other words, a particular supplement may be great for enhancing blood flow and at the same time may offer antimicrobial properties. (Most natural therapies offer multiple benefits—one of the great things about herbal medicine!) There are two basic forms of natural therapies: herbal medicine derived from plants, and bio-identical supplements.

Plant-Based Medicine

Plants must make a stand wherever the seed happens to land; tenacity is essential for survival. Tolerating harsh environmental conditions and fending off microbes of every variety is what they do; of course, some do it better than others. Our cultivated food plants have lost much of their survival abilities. Without being carefully tended, they quickly wither. For this reason, the medicinal value found in cultivated food plants is limited (so even the most healthful diet can carry you only so far). Plants used for herbal medicine, however, have very intense survival abilities. They are packed with chemical substances offering antioxidant, anti-inflammatory, anticancer, immune-enhancement, and broad-spectrum antimicrobial properties—all there for the benefit of the plant, but certainly, any creature that consumes the plant also gains the benefit.

Humans have known this for a very long time, and herbal medicine has always been a part of human culture (up until about 1930, when we exchanged herbs for drugs). The commonly used herbs typically have thousands of years of human use to their credit, so safety has been well-defined. Herbal therapies promote healing, and healing takes time; therefore, symptom reduction is generally much slower with herbs than drugs. Herbal therapies work best in synergy with combinations of multiple herbs, and often, high doses are required to gain maximal benefit (remember, herbs are more like a food substance than like a concentrated synthetic drug). Toxicity, however, is rarely a problem if the herbs are chosen carefully.

> Though herbs are not typically studied in the same fashion as drugs (and they shouldn't be, because they work differently), there is a very large body of scientific information available for most all of the commonly used herbal therapies. In fact, we probably know more about herbs than any other form of medicinal therapy (yes, even drugs; information about long-term use of most drugs is actually very limited), and accessing information about any herb on the planet is just a matter of doing an Internet search.

Bio-identical Supplements

Bio-identical supplements are the second category of natural therapy offering benefit for CF/FMS. These are natural substances that can be given to replace or enhance normal levels of identical chemical compounds in the human body. Vitamin C is a good example. The list includes vitamins, organic mineral compounds, amino acids, hormones such as estrogen and thyroid, and a host of other bioactive chemicals in the body.

The list can be further subdivided into essential and nonessential substances. "Essential" refers to substances that must be obtained from dietary sources to support human life (the body needs them but does not make them). This brief list includes vitamins, minerals, essential fatty acids, and nine essential amino acids (used for making proteins and certain chemical messengers in the body). Nonessential are the biochemical substances that the body normally makes (hormones, coenzyme Q10, glutathione, and many others).

With aging and disease, some nonessential substances can become essential. Insulin is essential for diabetics who have lost the capacity to produce insulin. Thyroid hormone replacement is important in someone suffering from thyroid disease. Coenzyme Q10 and the antioxidant glutathione decline with age and disease; replacement in CF/FMS can often be life-enhancing.

Notably, bio-identicals have been used therapeutically for less than a hundred years and are less well studied than any other medicinal therapy; there is still much to be learned about them, so they should be used cautiously and carefully. The potential for harm with bio-identicals is greater than commonly recognized, and bio-identicals are often used inappropriately. Though many bio-identical supplements are available commercially (and heavily promoted by the body-building industry and anti-aging doctors offering to replace all your hormones), the list of bio-identicals backed by good solid scientific evidence is rather short. The bio-identicals recommended in this book fall into that short list of substances with proven efficacy and safety.

TIPS ON TAKING SUPPLEMENTS

Please pay careful attention to the doses recommended, as any natural therapy must be dosed properly to give benefit. Often, the dose required to achieve efficacy is actually higher than that posted on the supplement label. Maximal benefit will, of course, be gained by synergy between multiple supplements, but you may want to start with just a few and work your way up.

When it comes to CF/FMS, one size does *not* fit all. The basic recommendations provided here may be quite adequate for someone with mild to moderate chronic fatigue, but someone with long-standing or severe CF/FMS will likely require a much more extensive regimen of supplements. Additional supplements are listed in Appendix B. A qualified healthcare provider can help guide your choices.

- **Be practical.** There are multiple ways of taking natural supplements, including fresh herbs, tinctures, teas, decoctions, tablets, powdered whole herbs, powdered extracts, and capsules. For most people, capsules work best. Capsules eliminate the bitter taste that comes with many supplements, and they keep well. They also travel well, as compared to other preparations. For practicality and convenience, capsules make sense; but accept that you will be taking a lot of capsules each day.

- **Stay organized.** By default, you end up with a bunch of different supplement bottles. It is convenient to keep them together in a shallow box such as a shoebox. Most supplements do not need to be refrigerated, so keeping them out on the counter (where you will see them and not forget them) is a good practice. Use a permanent marker to write on top of the bottle the number of capsules to be taken. Find a small cup (like a jigger glass) to put the capsules in before you take them. It is much easier to wash capsules down with a viscous liquid such as soy, almond, or coconut milk than with water. Eat something right after swallowing the capsules to make sure they go down.

- **Make it a habit.** Taking supplements needs to become a twice-daily ritual. In the beginning, put signs out, reminders, alarms, whatever it takes to get into the habit. Though dosing

3–4 times daily is often suggested as ideal, most people find that twice daily is about all they can handle. Therefore, the dosing recommendations I provide target twice-daily dosing: once in the morning and once in the evening. Taking your supplements should become such a firmly established habit that you feel like something is really missing if you forget.

- **Be a smart shopper.** Supplements can be taken as individual single-ingredient or combination supplements including several ingredients. The key to best results is proper dosing. Avoid supplements containing many ingredients (with the exception of multivitamin-type products); three to five ingredients should be the limit for combination therapeutic products. Avoid "proprietary blends," because the quantity of each individual ingredient is not stated (you really don't know what you are getting). There's a lot of hype out there; buy from a reputable source.

- **Start slowly.** Side effects with natural supplements are unusual, but they can occur. Start with only a few supplements at the lowest dose at first. This will help you define any side effects to a particular supplement. Start with one capsule of each supplement at a time. Gradually add others and increase the dose of each supplement. Synergy between supplements coupled with the proper therapeutic dose is generally required to achieve optimal benefit. Most supplements can be taken at the same time (unless otherwise specified).

- **Hang in there.** Often, people start feeling worse before they start feeling better. This is because supplements either kill microbes directly or restore the ability of the immune system to kill microbes. This will temporarily increase symptoms. In Lyme disease treatment, this phenomenon is referred to as a Herxheimer reaction, but it can occur with any microbial infection. If a new symptom occurs that can be specifically defined as a side effect to a particular supplement (such as nausea after taking a certain supplement), stop that supplement. If an exacerbation of **all** symptoms occurs, reduce the dose of **all** supplements until symptoms ease, and then gradually increase the dose over time again.

- **Make supplements part of your lifestyle.** Supplements to support general health can be continued indefinitely. Supplements that support immune function, reduce inflammation, and provide antimicrobial properties should be continued at the higher doses recommended until symptoms subside. At that point, doses can be reduced, but the supplements should not be discontinued completely. You will learn to rotate different assortments of supplements over time. Chronic fatigue recovery is a lifestyle, and natural supplements are an ongoing part of that lifestyle.

- **Check out the Quick List!** Descriptions are proved for each supplement in this chapter—you need to know something about what you are taking—but it does make for a long chapter. The summary at the end of the book provides a "quick list" of all the essential supplements for ease of use.

The natural supplements listed in this book have been carefully chosen for their very low potential for harm. Taking every single one of the supplements listed should cause no significant untoward effects. Though all of the herbs have similar properties (antimicrobial, anti-inflammatory, immune enhancement, antioxidant), taking multiple herbs provides synergy and comprehensive coverage. This helps cover all the bases and accelerates healing.

Contraindications are rare for any of the supplements listed, but if you are pregnant, are on blood thinners, or have any unusual medical concerns, you should consult a healthcare provider with knowledge of natural supplements before using any supplements.

Many people (I count myself as one of them) believe that the cure for every disease lies hidden in nature (and not in some patent office). If we were to invest as much money into understanding plant medicines as we are presently spending on new drugs, the world would be a better place. It doesn't, however, take a professional degree to learn about herbs and enjoy them. I invite you to explore the magic found in natural therapies, during your recovery and for the rest of your life!

PRIMARY SUPPLEMENTS FOR HEALING

The ingredients detailed in this chapter are very important for supporting natural healing processes in the body. They provide properties that restore energy to the body, reduce inflammation, restore normal immune function, and suppress low-virulence microbes. I have listed all ingredients separately with recommended dosing, so that supplements can be acquired from any reputable company. If you aren't sure where to start or would like to find combination supplements that offer therapeutic-doses of these ingredients, please visit https://vitalplan.com.

PROTECT MITOCHONDRIA AND BOOST ENERGY

Restoring energy and reducing fatigue is one of the most pressing concerns in CF/FMS. At the top of the list for restoring energy is protecting mitochondrial function, DNA, and cellular structures against free radicals, toxins, inflammatory processes, and pathogenic microbes. (For mitochondrial restoration, bio-identicals top the list, but herbal supplements will dominate most other categories.)

- **Alpha lipoic acid.** A potent antioxidant having the unique property of being both water- and fat-soluble. This enables it to be easily concentrated in blood, cells, tissues, and extracellular fluids (space and fluid between cells). It is easily absorbed and works with antioxidants already present inside cells to reduce cellular damage from free radicals. It also regenerates glutathione, the cell's most important antioxidant. Alpha lipoic acid enhances antioxidant effects of vitamin C, vitamin E, and NAC. It is protective of liver function and helps remove toxins from the body. It is also protective of nerve tissue and has been shown to reverse diabetic nerve damage. It enhances oxygenation of tissues, enhances immune function, and protects tissues against elevated glucose.

Suggested dosage: 250–300 mg twice daily.

Side effects: Rare.

- **Vitamin C.** Vitamin C provides almost too many functions in the body to list, but most important are antioxidant properties. When combined with other antioxidants, vitamin C offers a high degree of protection of tissues. Vitamin C is essential for collagen formation and is very important for chronic disease recovery. Vitamin C is concentrated in white blood cells. It offers antibacterial and antiviral properties. Vitamin C is inexpensive and should be considered a must-take supplement.

  Suggested dosage: 500–1000 mg twice daily during recovery. Lower doses are indicated after wellness is restored. Ascorbate is easier on the stomach.

  Side effects: Occasional gastric upset and loose stools at higher doses. If side effects occur, reduce the dose.

- **NAC (n-acetyl cysteine).** Another potent antioxidant, NAC is an essential component for formation of glutathione inside cells. NAC inhibits cytokine cascades (inflammatory messengers stimulated by microbes) and the breakdown of collagen. NAC concentrates in lungs and offers antioxidant effects and is mucolytic (breaks down mucus). It is strongly protective of nerve tissue. NAC also protects liver function. Combining therapeutic doses of lipoic acid, vitamin C, and NAC will raise glutathione levels inside cells better than will supplementing with glutathione.

Suggested dosage: 1000–2000 mg twice daily.

Side effects: Rare.

- **Coenzyme Q10 (CoQ10).** CoQ10 is an essential component of cellular energy production. CoQ10 is a key component of the machinery responsible for producing energy within mitochondria. Supplemental CoQ10 is another way to keep mitochondria humming, especially in organs requiring high energy such as the heart. Coenzyme Q10 also is a potent antioxidant that protects mitochondria. CoQ10 also inhibits free-radical damage to cell and mitochondrial membranes. The highest concentrations in the body are in the heart, liver, kidney, and pancreas. CoQ10 is especially protective of heart muscle.

  Suggested dosage: 50–100 mg twice daily (use Ubiquinol, the reduced form of CoQ10).

  Side effects: Rare.

REDUCE INFLAMMATION

Tissue/Vascular inflammation

Good blood flow is essential for healing to occur. Blood delivers oxygen and vital nutrients. Blood also removes toxic byproducts generated during exercise, and debris created by friction-damaged tissues or by injury. Blood flow, however, is often constricted by the inflammation that occurs with chronic disease—a toxic and vicious cycle. Chronic pain is the inevitable result. The supplements in this category reduce vascular inflammation and promote optimal blood flow.

- **Resveratrol from Japanese knotweed (JKW) (Polygonum cuspidatum).** Resveratrol is the age-defying substance found in grapes and wine that everybody is talking about. Grapes and wine, however, are not the only source of resveratrol.

Japanese knotweed (an herb from Asia naturalized to the United States) is a particularly good source of **trans**-resveratrol, the form most readily utilized by the body.

Resveratrol offers a list of benefits including potent antioxidant properties and support of normal heart function. It dilates blood vessels, improves blood flow, inhibits platelet aggregation (thins blood), and mildly lowers LDL cholesterol. Resveratrol is also protective of nerve tissue.

Beyond trans-resveratrol, the whole herb offers a spectrum of chemical substances that have medicinal value. Resveratrol and the whole herb support normal immune function and offer anti-inflammatory properties and anticancer properties. JKW is a double-duty supplement offering antimicrobial properties against many types of pathogenic bacteria and viruses. JKW has been used in traditional forms of Asian medicine for centuries and offers a high level of safety.

Suggested dosage: The commonly recommended dose of resveratrol for vascular benefit is 50–100 mg daily. The traditional dose of JKW and the dose of whole herb to achieve antimicrobial benefit is higher (See "Antimicrobials" below for proper dosage for antimicrobial benefit.)

Side effects: Rare. Low potential for toxicity.

- **French maritime pine bark (FMPB).** How pine trees native to the coast of France could have any bearing on your recovery is hard to imagine, but it is so. Potent antioxidants and other chemical compounds in FMPB inhibit platelet aggregation (blood thinner), reduce vascular inflammation, and improve the integrity of blood vessels. This improves blood flow to tissues; optimal blood flow is essential for recovering from CF/FMS. Potent anti-inflammatory properties also extend to offer protection for joints and ligaments. FMPB is also beneficial for the immune system.

Suggested dosage: 50–100 mg daily.

Side effects: Rare. Low potential for toxicity.

- **Hawthorn (Crataegus oxyacantha).** Hawthorn would be best described as a heart tonic. A tonic is a substance that has an overall positive effect on a particular organ system. For the heart, hawthorn meets the criteria. Hawthorn increases blood flow to the heart, strengthens contractions of the heart muscle, and improves circulation by dilating blood vessels. This allows increased oxygen delivery to tissues (very important for CF/FMS). It also reduces palpitations and provides a calming effect that reduces adrenaline. Hawthorn normalizes blood pressure. Hawthorn also lowers LDL cholesterol and has hypoglycemic activity in Type II diabetics.

  Suggested dosage: 500–1000 mg extract (combined leaf, stem, flower standardized to 1.8% Vitexin) twice daily. If any heart symptoms are present—palpitations, for example—hawthorn should be added to your supplement regimen.

  Side effects: Rare. Hawthorn is very safe for long-term use.

Joint and Tissue Inflammation

Joint pain and inflammation is a very common feature of CF/FMS. Reducing inflammation in joints and tissues is essential for recovery and damage control. The following supplements are well known for reducing arthritis-type inflammation. Unlike anti-inflammatory drugs, which inhibit healing as well as inflammation, natural herbs promote all aspects of healing along with reducing inflammation; therefore, they can safely be used long term (even for the rest of your life) without concern.

- **Turmeric (Curcuma longa).** Turmeric is the spice that defines an Indian curry. It may also be the reason why people of India have half the rate of cancer as we have here in the United States, and possibly the lowest rate of Alzheimer's in the world. A member of the ginger family, this herb offers potent anti-inflammatory properties and has a long history of use for arthritic conditions. It is known to inhibit multiple stages of cancer formation and has demonstrated well-proven anticancer properties in the lab. Extended use is associated with decreased dementia risk. Turmeric combines well with boswellia for synergistic effect. Turmeric protects liver cells, and unlike anti-inflammatory drugs, turmeric actually heals stomach ulcers.

Suggested dosage: Variable depending on the type of turmeric. Standardized extract 200–500 mg twice daily (depending on the type of extract used). High doses for arthritis are generally well tolerated. Absorption of the active chemicals is increased when turmeric is combined with black pepper extract (bioperine) or enzymes.

Side effects: Side effects are rare in turmeric's very long history of human use as both a food and a medicine.

- **Boswellia (Boswellia serrata).** Known in its native land as Indian frankincense, boswellia has been used for thousands of years for treatment of arthritic conditions. Offering potent anti-inflammatory properties, it is often combined with turmeric for treatment of arthritis and other inflammatory conditions. It is also known to inhibit the processes that lead to cancer.

  Suggested dosage: Variable depending on the supplement, but generally 150–300 mg twice daily.

  Side effects: Rare. Low potential for toxicity.

- **Devil's claw (Harpagophytum procumbens).** Native to southern Africa, devil's claw derives its name from hook-like appendages that cover the fruit of the plant. The "claws" attach to the fur of passing animals and distribute the seeds far and wide. The root of the plant is actually the part processed for medicine. Traditionally, devil's claw has been used for treatment of arthritic conditions and low-back pain. Use is supported by clinical studies.

Suggested dosage: 100–200 mg twice daily.

Side effects: Rare. Low potential for toxicity.

- **Glucosamine.** Glucosamine is a precursor for proteoglycans, the chemicals necessary for smooth and slick joint linings. It also stimulates synthesis of collagen, the base substance for cartilage. Glucosamine is formed by a molecule of glucose combined with the amino acid glutamine. With age, normal glucosamine synthesis decreases, which may be a contributing factor to arthritis.

  Suggested dosage: 500–750 mg twice daily.

  Side effects: Uncommon. Glucosamine HCl is derived from shellfish but does not contain the proteins that cause reactions in individuals with shellfish allergies. Studies have demonstrated that glucosamine HCl is well tolerated in people with shellfish allergies. Even so, if you have a shellfish allergy, use caution when taking glucosamine HCl. Presently, there is no evidence that glucosamine supplements appreciably affect blood glucose levels in diabetics.

- **Proteolytic digestive enzymes.** Enzymes that digest proteins are commonly present in many foods. These enzymes are known to be absorbed through the intestine into the bloodstream, where they have anti-inflammatory properties. Enzymes may play a role in removing damaged tissue (immune complexes). Some names of enzymes are familiar: bromelain from pineapple and papain from papaya. Protein-digesting enzymes play very important roles in not only reducing pain associated with arthritis but also reducing further damage of arthritis.

  Suggested use: Proteolytic enzymes, such as bromelain, are common ingredients in many arthritis formulas.

- **Vitamin C.** Essential for rebuilding cartilage (see above).

RESTORE IMMUNE FUNCTION

Compromised immune function is at the heart of all cases of CF/FMS. Pathogenic microbes like mycoplasma induce inflammation by stimulating chemical messengers called cytokines. Cytokines cause destructive inflammation that breaks down tissue. Symptoms of pain and fatigue are actually more closely related to cytokine stimulation than to direct damage caused by the microbe. The supplements in this category help reduce cytokines and also reduce inflammation. They normalize the immune response, allowing the immune system to properly deal with microbes and heal damage done by inflammation. At the same time, these supplements boost natural killer cells (NK cells), which are an important part of immune defense against intracellular microbes. They also offer some direct antimicrobial activity.

The herbs in this group are commonly referred to as adaptogens. Adaptogens are substances that restore balance in the face of stress. They reduce fatigue, restore normal immune function, balance central hormone pathways, and enhance the healing capacity of the body. Adaptogens are possibly the most important herbs for CF/FMS recovery.

- **Cordyceps (Cordyceps sinensis).** Native to Tibet, cordyceps is a fungal species that grows on a specific type of caterpillar during specific times of the year. Historically, its value was equal its weight to gold, and it was specifically reserved for emperors and royalty. Today, fortunately, high-quality cordyceps can be easily cultivated and its wonderful benefits are available to anyone.

  Cordyceps offers properties of immune enhancement and stress resistance. It protects mitochondria and is anti-fatigue. It is regularly used by Chinese and Russian athletes. In laboratory studies, cordyceps was found to reduce heart-muscle oxygen consumption and to improve aerobic activity. In traditional herbal medicine, it is often used as a kidney tonic.

Cordyceps specifically stimulates NK cells and macrophage activity and also enhances cellular immunity. At the same time, it decreases inflammatory cytokine cascades and therefore decreases tissue damage.

Suggested dosage: 1–3 grams (1000–3000 mg) cordyceps powder 2–3 times daily. (Some sources recommend 6–9 grams total per day as optimal.[8])

Side effects: Mild nausea can occur, but in general, side effects are rare, even with higher doses. Allergic reactions are rare.

- **Reishi (Ganoderma lucidum).** A mushroom with exceptional immune-modulating and antiviral properties. Reishi is a potent adaptogen. Extensively studied in Japan for potential anticancer properties, reishi mushrooms have been found to contain numerous potential cancer-fighting substances. Reishi offers important immune-modulation properties, reducing inflammatory cytokines and at the same time improving the response against threatening microbes and mutated cancer cells. It is calming and improves sleep. Anti-fatigue properties are related to restoration of normal adrenal-cortical function. It offers significant cardiovascular benefit and has been used to treat altitude sickness, suggesting that it may also increase oxygenation of tissues (a good thing because many intracellular pathogens thrive in a low-oxygen environment). Reishi is liver-protective.

Suggested dosage: 1–2 grams (1000–2000 mg) standardized extract (10%–14% polysaccharides) twice daily. (Higher dose range of 4 grams daily is recommended by some sources.[9])

Side effects: Extremely well tolerated, with rare side effects and no known toxicity.

---

[8] *Healing Lyme Disease Coinfections,* Stephen Harrod Buhner, Healing Arts Press, 2013.
[9] *Herbal Antivirals,* Stephen Harrod Buhner, Storey Publishing, 2013.

- **Rhodiola (Rhodiola rosea).** A favorite adaptogen of Russian athletes and workers for decreasing fatigue, increasing alertness, and improving memory, it is primarily sourced to Siberia, but different species of rhodiola grow worldwide. Though rhodiola is mildly stimulating, it restores natural sleep in the face of stress. Rhodiola offers antidepressant properties, providing a different option than St. John's wort (known for potential side effects). Rhodiola enhances cardiovascular function and immune function and protects nerve and brain tissue. Traditionally, rhodiola was used to improve work tolerance at high altitudes, and research suggests that it may increase oxygen delivery to tissues, especially the heart. Rhodiola also offers significant immune-modulating properties.

  Suggested dosage: 100–200 mg of standardized extract (2%–3% rosavins, 0.8%–1% salidroside) twice daily.

  Side effects: For some people, the herb is mildly stimulating. In general, however, rhodiola is well tolerated and is calming for most people.

- **Thymic extracts.** The thymus gland, located in the chest just behind the sternum, produces T-lymphocytes and immune-modulating substances vital for normal immune function. The most important of these substances is **thymic protein A (TPA)**. TPA orchestrates immune function by activating lymphocytes (white blood cells) for proper defense against viruses, bacteria, and other harmful agents.

  By age 40, the thymus gland has begun to atrophy, and loss of thymic function is a key factor in immune deficiency that occurs with aging and disease.

  Supplementation with TPA can dramatically improve immune function in immune-compromised individuals. Anyone demonstrating compromised immune function, chronic infections, chronic fatigue, low white blood cell count, or chronic exposure to toxins can potentially gain benefit. Thymic extracts have also been found to be beneficial for allergic rhinitis, asthma, and food sensitivities. TPA may also benefit autoimmune disorders, recurrent bacterial and viral infections, and some cancers (breast, for example). Even healthy individuals over age 50 can benefit with a maintenance dose of TPA for increased vitality and longevity.

The most reliable form of thymic extract, thymic protein A (ProBoost) is made in a laboratory from cell cultures and not by extraction from animal byproducts. Route of supplementation is sublingual (under the tongue), avoiding degradation by stomach acid. Supplementation is considered very safe with few side effects.

Suggested dosage: 1–3 packets of ProBoost daily until normal health is restored (for at least a month or two).

Side effects: Rare. Well tolerated.

- **Vitamin D.** The "sunshine vitamin" is important for more than just healthy bones. Vitamin D is essential for too many functions in the body to mention, but it is especially important for normal immune function. If adequate levels of vitamin D are not present in the body, normal immune function cannot occur. Vitamin D is created in the skin with exposure to UV rays of sunlight. Because much of the population works indoors and liberally applies sunscreen when going outside, low vitamin D levels have become very common. Aging and chronic disease also seem to adversely affect the ability of the body to generate vitamin D from sunlight. Though the best source of vitamin D is sunlight, supplementation is often necessary.

Suggested dosage: Full sun exposure, best between 10 a.m. and 2 p.m., is best for generating vitamin D. Thirty minutes to an hour every day to the arms, chest, and face without sunscreen is generally adequate. The way to know for sure is by having your vitamin D levels checked. During the winter months especially, supplements are the only way to gain adequate levels. People living in southern locations generally need 1000–2000 IU daily, whereas people in northern locations often require 4000 IU or greater. Dark-skinned people also often require larger amounts of vitamin D. Vitamin D_3 is the preferred form of supplementation. Again, the best way to know for sure is by having your vitamin D levels checked regularly (about every 3–6 months is ideal). Target a level of >40 ng/ml.

A combination of cordyceps, reishi, and rhodiola is beneficial for general chronic fatigue, mycoplasma infections, and viral infections. Eleuthero (see below) is especially beneficial for Lyme disease. All four can be used together, or they can be taken independently. Thymic extracts are expensive but should be considered for use early on to accelerate restoration of immune function. And, of course, restoration of normal immune function is not possible without adequate levels of vitamin D.

SUPPRESS PATHOGENS

Herbal antimicrobials are not as potent as conventional prescription antibiotics, but they do offer some distinct advantages in treatment of intracellular pathogens. Conventional antibiotics target one weak spot of a specific microbe with a single chemical agent. This limits range of therapy and opens the door for resistance to occur—any pathogen exposed to an antibiotic long enough will eventually develop resistance to that antibiotic.

Herbs with antimicrobial properties typically contain a wide spectrum of active chemical compounds; therefore, occurrence of microbial resistance is uncommon. Instead of being lethal to the microbe, herbal antimicrobials suppress growth and generally make the life of the microbe miserable enough for the immune system to gain ground.

Herbs also enhance immune function and promote healing in other ways. Because the toxicity of herbs is so low, they can be used at high concentrations for extended periods without concern.

Especially when it comes to dealing with intracellular pathogens, herbal antimicrobials are the best tool for the job. (Conventional antibiotics and herbs with antimicrobial properties can be used together for a synergistic effect.)

- **Resveratrol from Japanese knotweed (Polygonum cuspidatum).** Truly a wonder substance, Japanese knotweed is mentioned here again for its exceptional antimicrobial activity. Japanese knotweed is active against a wide range of bacterial pathogens. It is a primary herbal for both Lyme disease and mycoplasma treatment. Antiviral and antifungal properties are also present. Note that recommended dosages to suppress pathogens are higher than those used for purely vascular benefit.

  Very important general antimicrobial for Lyme, mycoplasma, general CF/FMS, and viral infections.

  Suggested dosage: 1–4 200 mg capsules Japanese knotweed (standardized to 50% trans-resveratrol) twice daily. Work up to 4 capsules twice daily until symptoms are resolving, and then gradually reduce back to 1 capsule twice daily.

  Side effects: Rare, with low potential for toxicity. Caution is advised if also taking anticoagulants, because resveratrol has blood-thinning properties.

- **Chinese skullcap (Scutellaria baicalensis).** Chinese skullcap is a potent synergist (increases benefit of other supplements), a property that is very important when choosing a supplement regimen. In other words, it enhances the value of other herbs, especially those with antimicrobial value. It is, by itself, strongly antiviral (especially against herpes viruses). It also offers antibacterial and antifungal properties. It is one of the primary supplements for use against mycoplasma. Chinese skullcap is also known for sedative properties. It contains melatonin, helpful for inducing sleep, and is strongly protective of nerve tissue. It also attenuates (calms) overactive immune function.

Chinese skullcap is an important synergist for mycoplasma and antiviral protocols.

Suggested dosage: 1 gram (1000 mg) 2–3 times daily. Use only the root extract, preferably 3-year plant with pronounced yellow color. (American skullcap does not offer the same antimicrobial properties and should not be substituted.)

Side effects: Rare, even at high doses, and are mostly gastrointestinal.

Taking high doses of herbal supplements long term can occasionally cause an upset stomach. If this occurs, you should take a break from the herbal therapy until the upset resolves. Drinking ginger tea several times a day will help settle your stomach and resolve any gastric inflammation present. Ginger also offers excellent antiviral and anti-inflammatory properties. To make ginger tea, buy fresh gingerroot from the grocery. Peal a thumb-sized piece and chop it up. Place in a tea strainer or in the bottom of a coffee cup. Pour in water heated to boiling temperature. Steep in the cup for several minutes. Add honey to sweeten, and drink up!

Additional Antimicrobial Support for Lyme Disease

If Lyme disease has been documented or is highly suspected, the following herbal therapies should be added to the daily regimen. The recommendations are in line with those made by Stephen Buhner in *Healing Lyme*. Thousands of patients have followed his protocol with exceptional results. If you have Lyme disease, I would strongly recommend reading the book. Having Lyme disease, however, certainly does not exclude the presence of other microbes. Note that all of these herbs are broad-spectrum and have activity against other bacteria and viruses.

- **Japanese knotweed.** Ditto to everything mentioned so far, and also considered a primary supplement for Lyme disease!

- **Eleuthero (Eleutherococcus senticosus).** Also known as Siberian ginseng, eleuthero has been used for thousands of years to fight infections and increase quality of life. Strongly stimulates the immune system. It offers similar properties to rhodiola, and the two can be used together or interchangeably; eleuthero, however, may have more potent antiviral and antibacterial properties. Adaptogenic, eleuthero improves stress resistance in all systems of the body. It restores normal adrenal function and normalizes immune function in the face of stress. It is protective against radiation and is liver-protective.

  Suggested dosage: 1:1 tincture (Russian extraction) from the root, 1 teaspoon twice daily (the second dose should be taken early in the afternoon to prevent evening stimulation). Dried herb extracts: 500 mg twice daily. Extracts from the Siberian region of Russia or extracts grown in America are generally preferred to extracts obtained from China.

  Side effects: Eleuthero tends to be more stimulating than rhodiola but is still not as stimulating as Panax ginseng. For most people, the herb is very well tolerated with a low potential for toxicity. Traditionally, eleuthero is taken for long periods of time.

- **Cat's claw (Uncaria tomentosa).** Native to the Amazon, cat's claw has a long history of traditional use for treatment of a wide range of inflammatory conditions. It also has been adopted by the Lyme community as a primary herb for use in Lyme disease. It offers immune-enhancing properties and potent anti-inflammatory properties. It is known to increase white blood cells, including B and T lymphocytes, natural killer (NK) cells, and granulocytes. Cat's claw is also known to enhance a specific type of NK cell, called CD57, which is deficient in Lyme disease. Cat's claw has anti-inflammatory and antimicrobial properties and has demonstrated healing properties for the GI tract.

Cat's claw is a primary herbal for Lyme disease and gastrointestinal restoration.

Suggested dosage: 1–4 400–500 mg capsules of 10:1 concentrate inner bark 2–3 times daily. It is especially important to take this herb with food, as it is activated by stomach acid. If you take acid-blocking drugs, cat's claw will have limited value.

Side effects: Occasional stomach upset, but generally very well tolerated.

- **Andrographis (Andrographis paniculata).** Another important herb from India, andrographis offers antiviral, antibacterial, and antiparasitic properties. It is widely used in the treatment of Lyme disease. Beyond Lyme disease, numerous clinical trials have demonstrated the ability of andrographis to reduce the length and severity of common viral illnesses. It has shown activity against viral hepatitis B and C. Andrographis has been used for dysentery and shows activity against pathogenic strains of E. coli. It is active against common roundworms and tapeworms. In a 2011 study, andrographis was found to be beneficial for ulcerative colitis. Additional benefits include immune enhancement and cardio-protective effects. Andrographis also offers significant liver protection.

Andrographis is an excellent antiviral and is important for Lyme disease and for gastrointestinal restoration.

Suggested dosage: 1–4 400mg capsules, extract standardized to 10% andrographolides twice daily.

Side effects: About 1% of people who take andrographis develop an allergic reaction, with whole-body hives and itching skin. The reaction will resolve gradually over several weeks after stopping use of the herb.

- **Sarsaparilla (Smilax glabra).** Sarsaparilla is native to South America, but Smilax species with medicinal benefit are common around the world. The most important property of sarsaparilla is its ability to bind endotoxins. Endotoxins are the

debris created when pathogenic bacteria are killed off. Endotoxins cause pain and fatigue and are the root of Herxheimer
reactions.

Sarsaparilla also offers antibacterial and antifungal properties.
It is commonly used in Lyme disease protocols. Traditionally,
it is used for treatment of psoriasis and other skin conditions.
Also, sarsaparilla has also been used traditionally for treatment of syphilis (another spirochete, like borrelia). Sarsaparilla increases bioavailability of other herbs and enhances
benefit (it is a synergist). Other beneficial properties include
potent anti-inflammatory and antioxidant properties. Sarsparilla enhances immune function.

*Sarsparilla is an important synergist for Lyme protocols and is
important for restoration of gastrointestinal function.*

Suggested dosage: 1–3 400–500 mg capsules of root extract
twice daily.

Side effects: Uncommon. Sarsaparilla is generally well tolerated.

- **Allisure® garlic (Allium sativum).** Allisure® is a patented
  extract of stabilized garlic. Garlic has been used as a medicinal
  since the beginning of recorded time, but the active chemicals
  in garlic, called acillins, are very volatile. The smell of crushed
  garlic is acillin; it dissipates as soon as the garlic is crushed,
  cooked, or consumed. Less than 1% is actually absorbed in
  active form; therefore, benefit from standard garlic preparations is highly variable and often minimal.

  A company from the UK has successfully stabilized acillin so
  that yield is increased to nearly 100%. The product, called
  Allisure®, has been shown to have potent broad-spectrum
  activity against gram-positive and gram-negative bacteria, as
  well as having antiviral, antifungal, and antiparasitic properties.

  Allisure® has demonstrated activity against MRSA infections.
  Lyme disease patients have noted significant benefit. Allisure®

is highly beneficial for chronic fungal infections and shows remarkable cardiovascular benefits. It lowers cholesterol, inhibits platelet aggregation (stickiness), improves blood flow, reduces blood pressure, and has direct cardiogenic effects.

Allisure® is an excellent general antimicrobial and is excellent for gastrointestinal restoration.

Suggested dosage: 180–360 mg 2–3 times daily.

Side effects: Extremely well tolerated. The estimated toxic dose is 3000 capsules per day!

CONVENTIONAL MEDICAL OPTIONS

Pharmaceuticals can be useful in the management of CF/FMS but should be reserved for specific indications because of the potential for side effects and toxicity. The addictive potential of certain drugs should be respected. All synthetic drugs are potential poisons and should be respected as such. Drugs are the most toxic of all therapies, and chronic use should be limited to the lowest dose to achieve benefit. Many medications have the potential to cause vitamin and mineral deficiencies.

That being said, drugs can ease symptoms acutely and can slow destructive processes associated with inflammatory disease. In the larger scheme of things, this can be very important. Using drugs in a constructive fashion is a matter of

- using the lowest dose possible to elicit a positive response,

- using the drug for only as long as necessary,

- combining drug therapy with appropriate natural supplements to maximize healing, and

- using drugs with potential for addiction only intermittently and only when necessary.

Of all classes of drugs, conventional antibiotics have the most direct positive influence on the healing process. Different types of antibiotics are designed to kill or inhibit bacteria, viruses, fungi, and protozoa. Acutely, this can have great benefit. Prolonged use, however, generally results in antibiotic resistance, suppression of immune function, and disruption of normal gut flora.

Find a healthcare provider who understands the potential toxicity of drugs and knows how to administer them properly as part of a comprehensive strategy of health restoration.

The following list is meant for informational purposes only. It is provided to help you better understand medications you may already be taking or that a healthcare provider may recommend. It is not meant to dictate therapy or to suggest in any way that you should be taking these drugs.

Immune/Antimicrobial

- **Conventional antibiotic therapy.** For CF/FMS, antibiotics are mostly useful for acute infections in which the offending microbe can be well defined. Benefit declines exponentially the longer an antibiotic is used; antibiotic resistance, immune suppression, and disruption of normal gut flora limit chronic use. Also, the pathogenic microbes associated with CF/FMS are generally intracellular, where conventional antibiotics have limited benefit.

- **Fluconazole.** The standard conventional drug treatment for chronic yeast is fluconazole 150 mg weekly for as long as six months. This regimen, however, like many conventional therapies, does not address the cause. Also, fluconazole-resistant yeast is becoming more of a concern. Fluconazole is indicated for only short-term treatment when Candida has been definitively diagnosed. Most chronic yeast infections will resolve as normal health is restored.

- **Systemic steroids.** Sustained high doses of steroids strongly suppress immune function. Although this is sometimes necessary to suppress a destructive inflammatory process, steroids also inhibit the normal healing processes in the body. Long-term use is associated with gastric erosions, insomnia, weight gain, increased risk of infections, and a long list of other potential side effects. Systemic steroids (oral, intravenous, intramuscular) should be used for the shortest duration possible to achieve benefit. Natural supplements will decrease the need for long-term steroid use.

Prednisone, prednisolone, and cortisone are the most commonly used oral steroids.

- **Immune drugs.** Immune drugs selectively inhibit specific portions of the immune system. This is the newest tactic offered by the pharmaceutical industry for treating autoimmune disease. Although these drugs are more specific than steroids, they are still part of the old approach of fixing the process approach instead of addressing the causes. It perpetuates "managed illness" and dependence on the drug (drug companies would go out of business if they designed drugs that actually cured disease). Humira and Remicade are two immune drugs. All increase risk of certain types of infection and cancer. Although these drugs do have value, use should be limited to severe cases in which there is no other choice. (They are certainly not the panacea often conveyed by the commercials.)

- **Valcyte (valganciclovir).** Valcyte is an antiviral specific for herpes-type viruses, especially indicated for CMV infection. Diagnosing a flare-up of CMV or other herpes-type viruses is challenging, but CF/FMS patients have gained benefit from arbitrary use of Valcyte during a flare-up of symptoms. Muscle pain associated with flu-like symptoms would be best expected to respond. The potential for harm with arbitrary use is low.

- **IV-Ig (intravenous antibody therapy).** IV injections of immunoglobulin have been studied for use in treatment of chronic fatigue syndromes, but to date, there has been no evidence that IV-Ig has any effect on chronic fatigue.

MEDICAL PROCEDURES

Beyond drugs and natural therapies are medical procedures—things done to you. Conventional medical procedures include steroid (and other drug) injections into joints, joint replacements, and pain-management procedures such as epidurals. Though medical procedures do have the ability to restore function, expense and associated risks are high.

These procedures should be reserved for use when cumulative damage has compromised function beyond the restorative capacity of the body. They should not be first-line therapies or go-to therapies prior to the other options mentioned first. The risk of complications such as immune suppression or infection cannot be overstated. Reducing inflammation with herbals is very important prior to undergoing some procedures and may improve outcomes.

The therapies discussed in this section are designed to tap into the healing processes of the body and to slow destructive processes of disease, but initially, they may have little effect on reducing symptoms. Healing takes time, and symptoms do not go away until healing is well underway. The next chapter is therefore devoted to addressing the two most uncomfortable symptoms of CF/FMS: pain and sleep disturbances.

CHAPTER 6

SYMPTOM CONTROL: PAIN AND SLEEP

Fatigue is the most predominant symptom associated with CF/FMS, but chronic pain and trouble sleeping are the most disturbing and uncomfortable of all symptoms possible. As healing occurs, these and other symptoms will gradually resolve, but in the short term, addressing pain and poor sleep is important for your recovery to move in a positive direction.

PAIN, A CARDINAL FEATURE OF CF/FMS

Focusing on getting better is a real challenge when pain gets in the way. Pain is a daily aggravation that inhibits sleep and slows recovery. Reducing the symptom of pain can be as important as reducing the causes of pain. Though the mechanisms of pain are complex and still being sorted out, knowing the basics of why pain occurs can help formulate a plan for reducing pain.

Pain receptors occur in all tissues and organs in the body. The highest concentrations of receptors are in the skin—pain is felt more specifically in skin than anywhere else. When pain receptors are stimulated, the impulse is conducted by different types of nerves and is "felt" in different areas of the brain. The degree of stimulation and number of receptors activated define the intensity of pain. Acute pain is typically caused by trauma and is felt differently than chronic pain caused by inflammation and nerve damage.

The simple act of moving about creates friction where ligaments and joints rub against one another. This minor trauma stimulates pain receptors. If it were not for powerful pain-inhibiting chemicals called endorphins circulating in the body, you wouldn't be able to get up off the couch. Endorphins make normal movement possible. In addition to relieving pain, they also promote feelings of well-being and play an important role in enhancing immune function. Ya gotta have endorphins to survive!

If tissues are healthy, endorphins completely suppress the perception of pain associated with normal movement, but if tissues are inflamed or damaged, the perception of pain breaks through. Inflammation of muscles, joints, ligaments, and other tissues is the root cause of chronic pain in CF/FMS. When muscles become chronically inflamed, spasm or twitch occurs. This, of course, increases pain but also places undue pressure at certain points (these are the trigger points of fibromyalgia). Chronic stress (of any type) suppresses normal endorphin production. Not surprisingly, CF/FMS is associated with high inflammation and low endorphins.

STRATEGIES FOR ADDRESSING PAIN

Drugs are sometimes the only solution for pain control. The potency of drugs is sometimes necessary to control pain. If they are used properly, drugs can positively support the healing process. The key is using them properly. Non-narcotic pharmaceuticals are preferred when long-term use of a medication is required. Narcotic pain relievers should be reserved exclusively for acute pain and should never be used long term.

The role of natural supplements is mainly supportive. Healing is the most important quality offered by natural supplements. Their value for controlling the symptom of pain is really very limited. Even so, the potential for harm is extremely low, and use of natural supplements can reduce the need for prescription medications. All of the frequently cited natural supplements offering potential pain reduction are listed below. Some, however, offer only minimal value—this is noted in each case.

Alternative therapies also offer important support. Acupuncture, massage therapy, and other alternative therapies not only support the healing process but also can reduce pain directly.

The ultimate solution for chronic pain is reducing inflammation. Initially, anti-inflammatory drugs can be beneficial for slowing or stopping destructive processes, but side effects limit long-term use. Natural anti-inflammatory substances (herbs and bio-identical natural supplements) are not as potent as the drugs, but you can use them for a lifetime with no worries. Drugs and natural anti-inflammatory supplements can be safely started at the same time and used together. The drugs can usually be discontinued after the healing process is underway.

Raising endorphin levels is one of the primary keys to getting well. Having normal endorphin levels is intimately tied to good health and well-being. Baseline secretion of endorphins can be increased with regular exercise, vigorous massage, and acupuncture. Orgasm and consumption of spicy food (hot peppers) also increase endorphin secretion. Chronic stress decreases endorphins, and not surprisingly, regular practice of meditation or relaxation techniques stimulates endorphins. Just having a warm, friendly attitude will also increase endorphins. Novel ways of increasing endorphin production include administration of very low doses of a drug called naltrexone and use of human chorionic gonadotropin (see "Novel Pharmaceutical Applications" below).

Food sensitivities are often the source of muscle pain and fatigue associated with CF/FMS. Often, multiple foods are involved. Sensitivities to wheat products, soy, tree nuts, peanuts, and potatoes are common, but sensitivities to any foods can occur. Generally, the more commonly consumed foods are at fault. Food sensitivities can change over time as foods are rotated, but the good news is that food sensitivities generally improve or resolve with restoration of normal immune function. In the short term, however, avoidance is the best policy. Food sensitivities can be defined with a food sensitivity testing panel or an elimination diet. (Both are sometimes a good idea if multiple food sensitivities are suspected.) An elimination diet is provided in chapter 8, "Purify."

Unrelenting pain should, of course, be brought to the attention of your healthcare provider. Pain associated with other symptoms is more concerning than isolated pain by itself. For example, abdominal pain with vomiting or fever is generally much more

*concerning than isolated abdominal pain alone (though severe
pain at any location, especially abdominal, should be brought to
the attention of a healthcare provider).*

NATURAL CHOICES FOR PAIN RELIEF

- **Natural anti-inflammatory supplements.** Natural substances with anti-inflammatory and pain-relieving properties
  include **boswellia, devil's claw, turmeric, ginger, MSM,** and
  glucosamine. These supplements should be considered
  essential for reducing inflammation that causes pain. **Chinese
  skullcap** also has a history of offering benefit for reducing
  pain. These are all primary supplements discussed in the pre-
  vious chapter.

- **Cherries.** Cherries contain chemicals with anti-inflammatory
  properties and pain-relieving qualities—about 10–12 fresh or
  dried cherries several times daily can help reduce pain. Fresh,
  dried, or frozen, enjoy them whenever you can!

- **Systemic enzyme therapy.** Supplemental enzymes are most
  commonly used to facilitate digestion of food but can also
  relieve inflammation and reduce pain. Protein-digesting
  enzymes break down immune complexes that are part of the
  inflammatory process. Common protein-digesting enzymes
  found in supplements include **bromelain** from pineapple and
  papain from papaya. You could eat lots of pineapple and
  papaya, but a better option is taking a standard digestive
  enzyme supplement with meals.

- **Sarsaparilla.** Pain can be associated with endotoxins produced by dying bacteria. The source can be from die-off of bacteria during treatment of Lyme disease (Herxheimer reaction)
  or from buildup of abnormal bacteria in the gut. Either way,
  sarsaparilla binds and removes endotoxins and therefore can
  aid in reducing pain. Sarsaparilla is discussed as a primary
  herb in chapter 5, "Enhance Healing."

- **Black cohosh (Cimicifuga racemosa).** Black cohosh is
  excellent for relieving deep muscular pain and body aches

worsened by cold. Traditionally used mostly for rheumatism, black cohosh also offers anti-inflammatory properties. Also beneficial for reducing nerve pain.

Suggested dosage: 40–80 mg of standardized extract daily.

Side effects: well tolerated.

- **St. John's wort (Hypericum perforatum).** St. John's wort naturally increases serotonin. Serotonin is considered the "mood" hormone but is also tied to pain pathways. Low serotonin is associated with chronic pain. Increasing serotonin with St. John's wort or drug therapy can benefit both mood and pain perception. (See also Cymbalta under drug therapy.)

Suggested dosage: Dependent on supplement chosen.

Side effects: St. John's wort can adversely affect concomitant drug therapy.

- **D-phenylalanine.** D-phenylalanine is an essential amino acid often marketed for pain relief. Typically, high doses are recommended. There are no studies, however, showing positive efficacy. This one is probably best left on the shelf.

- **Topical capsaicin or menthol.** Topical application (creams, rubs, and patches) is effective for local pain such as muscle strain or low-back pain. Application of capsaicin is thought to reduce "substance P" (we don't know what substance P is yet, but we do know it has to be present for local pain to occur). Use of capsaicin is limited by irritation of skin. Menthol has a cooling effect that decreases perception of pain.

- **Animal venom.** Different types of venom are being studied for interrupting nerve pathways associated with pain. Right now, there are two primary venom products on the market: bee venom (different producers) and cobra venom (Nyloxin). Both are effective for reducing pain, but potential side effects from blocking other nerve pathways are still being deciphered. Preparations can be applied topically for local pain or taken sublingually (under the tongue) for systemic pain. Side effects with local use are uncommon, but systemic use is associated with reducing gastrointestinal mobility, thus causing nausea.

♦ **Bee venom** is a natural product that has been used for ages with documented benefit for arthritis.

♦ **Nyloxin** is an FDA-approved over-the-counter pharmaceutical that uses standardized doses of cobra venom for use in controlling moderate pain.

- **Exercise.** Regular exercise increases natural endorphins.

- **Deep relaxation.** Regular practice of meditation or deep relaxation increases endorphins and decreases pain. These practices can also reduce the perception of pain and the anxiety that comes with it.

- **Deep heat.** A warm bath or a heating pad applied to specific areas can help soothe muscular pain.

The slow continuous movements and gentle stretching associated with yoga and Qigong are ideally suited for CF/FMS recovery. Regular practice not only improves mobility but also helps relieve pain. Not only are these ancient Eastern practices simple to learn, but anybody of almost any level of fitness can do them. Qigong is the easier of the two, but yoga is more well-known. Yoga classes are everywhere, and basic Qigong can be easily picked up from watching YouTube videos.

PHARMACEUTICALS FOR PAIN MANAGEMENT

- **Cymbalta.** This antidepressant increases both serotonin and norepinephrine in the brain and offers significant benefit for relief of muscle pain. Use is limited by worsening of insomnia in some patients. Taken once daily, 30–60 mg.

- **Neurontin (gabapentin).** Gabapentin is an anti-seizure drug effective for treatment of symptoms associated with nerve damage. It is useful for control of pain associated with CF/FMS and other nerve-related symptoms. It can also be useful for sleep. Common side effects include sedation, dizziness, dry mouth, and constipation. Side effects increase as the dosage is increased. Tolerance may develop over time. Taken 3 times daily.

- **Lyrica (pregabalin).** Similar to Neurontin, Lyrica is effective for relief of symptoms associated with nerve damage and is useful for control of pain associated with CF/FMS and other nerve-related symptoms. Common side effects include sedation, dizziness, dry mouth, and constipation. Tolerance may develop. Taken 3 times daily.

- **Nonsteroidal anti-inflammatory medications (NSAIDs).** NSAIDs provide anti-inflammatory benefit and relief from mild pain. Chronic use is limited by risk of inducing stomach ulcers and increased risk of cardiovascular disease. Ibuprofen and naproxen are primary examples. Mobic (meloxicam) is a newer-generation NSAID that has to be taken only once daily.

- **NSAID topical creams.** NSAIDs can be compounded into topical creams to be applied directly to painful joints and muscles. Local application decreases gastric irritation.

- **Toradol (ketoprofen).** Toradol is an anti-inflammatory drug with pain and anti-inflammatory action that is in the same class as ibuprofen but is much more potent. Toradol is administered by injection intramuscularly (IM) or intravenously (IV). It is also available as a nasal spray. Use is generally limited to the short term because of potential long-term side effects.

- **Tylenol (acetaminophen).** Acetaminophen should be avoided because of potential liver compromise.

- **Narcotic medications (opioids).** Opioid medications control pain by mimicking natural endorphins. They are very effective for acute pain, but chronic use is associated with habituation and addiction. Chronic use actually lowers pain tolerance because it suppresses natural endorphins. Chronic use should be avoided if at all possible! Common narcotics include morphine, Demerol, Dilaudid, Percocet (oxycodone/acetaminophen), Vicodin (hydrocodone/acetaminophen), and many others.

- **Ultram (tramadol).** This novel pain medication has opiate-like characteristics but is less sedating and less addictive than opioids. The potential for tolerance and dependence, however, exists with continuous use. Excessive use does suppress natural endorphins.

- **Muscle relaxers (Soma, Flexeril).** Muscle relaxers are indicated only for short-term relief of chronic muscular pain associated with spasm. The mechanism of action of muscle relaxers is not completely understood (as with so many drugs), but these drugs have sedative actions on the peripheral and central nervous system. Chronic use of muscle relaxers is associated with habituation, dependence, and withdrawal symptoms.

- **Steroid injections.** Cortisone injections into inflamed joints reduce pain and inflammation, but frequent or chronic use can increase atrophy of tissues.

- **Lidocaine patches.** Local anesthetics numb tissues, but when they are injected, the relief does not last very long. Patches slowly release the local anesthetic to provide longer relief.

For acute pain or severe pain unrelieved by other measures, most people end up taking narcotics (morphine and morphine-like drugs). The pain-relieving properties offered by these drugs are more potent than any other substances on earth. Narcotics work quite well, and when there is no other reasonable choice, use of them can be lifesaving. Long-term use (any longer than a month or two), however, quickly leads to habituation and addiction. Because narcotics are so heav-ily prescribed, America has developed a serious opioid prob-lem: 80% of the world's opioid supply is consumed by Americans, mostly by prescription.

NOVEL PHARMACEUTICAL APPLICATIONS

- **Low-dose naltrexone (LDN).** LDN is a novel therapy for chronic pain and immune dysfunction. Naltrexone, a drug designed to block the effects of narcotics, when used in very low doses (4.5 mg as compared to the standard therapeutic dose of 50 mg) causes the body to produce high levels of nat-ural endorphins. Low-dose naltrexone therapy appears to be safe and free of significant short-term or long-term side effects. Naltrexone is a prescription drug. Lower doses must be formulated by a compounding pharmacy. In many cases, low-dose naltrexone obviates the need for any other drug therapy. **Users must be completely free of all narcotic med-ications for at least 2 weeks before using naltrexone.** See lowdosenaltrexone.org for information.

- **Human Chorionic Gonadotropin (HCG).** HCG is a peptide (protein-like) hormone produced in early pregnancy that mimics other brain-stem hormones. It primarily affects the hypothalamus, the area of the brain that regulates weight, temperature, night and day cycles, and other automatic func-tions. Very low doses of HCG have been utilized in weight loss programs around the world for sixty years. It is reported to be effective and the reported incidence of side effects is very low.

Interestingly, many patients with CF/FMS and autoimmune conditions using HCG for weight loss have reported decreased pain and improvement in other symptoms. This seems to be a repeatable phenomenon and physicians caring primarily for fibromyalgia patients have taken notice. HCG is now being used by some fibromyalgia clinics. HCG must be obtained by prescription from a healthcare provider.

No one knows exactly why HCG works for weight loss or reducing pain, but it is theorized to enhance endorphin production. Endorphins are produced by the hypothalamus and pituitary gland. HCG mildly stimulates the hypothalamus. Mild stimulation of the hypothalamus by HCG may increase endorphin secretion.

- **Medical marijuana.** Though still quite controversial, medical marijuana may hold great promise for CF/FMS sufferers. Most users experience significantly reduced pain, better sleep, and improved sense of well-being. Marijuana is habituating, but risk of use appears to be far less than narcotics or other drugs. Where legal, medical marijuana should be used under supervision of a qualified healthcare provider. Intermittent use is preferred. Use by inhalation should be avoided. Marijuana is primarily beneficial for symptom reduction and should not be considered a substitute for other healing therapies.

ALTERNATIVE AND COMPLEMENTARY THERAPIES

Credibility can be an issue with some alternative therapies and some alternative therapy providers. Before choosing an alternative therapy, search the Internet for scam reports about that particular therapy. Although most alternative therapies have a low potential for harm, some could still be a waste of your money. The same is true with alternative therapy providers; if the price seems too high or if therapy obligates you for many visits, do some investigation before laying your money down.

- **Massage therapy.** A skilled massage therapist can do wonders for body aches and muscle pain. Ask around to find someone with experience working with CF/FMS patients. Massage can reduce symptoms and also generate natural endorphins.

- **Physical therapy.** Stiffness in joints, ligaments, and muscles is almost a given in CF/FMS. Physical therapy can help restore the body back to normal.

- **Acupuncture.** Standard acupuncture reduces symptoms, restores energy flow in the body, increases endorphins, and can result in long-term improvement.

- **Chiropractic care.** Manipulations performed by a skilled chiropractor can effectively reduce musculoskeletal pain.

- **Frequency-specific acupuncture.** Possibly the most intriguing alternative therapy for CF/FMS is frequency-specific acupuncture. Specific frequency electrical micro-current is applied to acupuncture needles placed at key locations around the body. The electrical frequencies are "tuned" to the types of microbes common in CF/FMS. The procedure can also be performed with specific frequency light-emitting diodes (LEDs) instead of acupuncture needles. Acupuncture is complemented with homeopathic remedies specific to the microbes. In this fashion, targeted microbes are eliminated and immune function is restored. Though the science to back it up is limited, the potential for harm is low. The chief obstacle is cost—plan on spending $600–$2000 for a complete course of therapy.

- **Energy medicine.** Some people have remarkably positive experiences with energy medicine, but results are highly variable. The primary benefit is reduction in pain and other symptoms; complete restoration of health should not be expected.

MEDICAL PROCEDURES FOR PAIN MANAGEMENT

- **Transcutaneous electrical nerve stimulation (TENS).** TENS reduces pain by interrupting irritation nerve impulses associated with muscle spasm and twitches. It is effective for mild to moderate muscular pain. A TENS unit can be purchased without a prescription from pharmacies and the Internet. Risk of use and side effects are very low.

- **Oxygen therapy.** It has been proposed that intensive oxygen intake through breathing pure oxygen or spending time in a hyperbaric oxygen chamber could improve recovery of CF/FMS, but studies have not shown significant benefit. There are reports, however, of improvement in neuropathies (tingling and burning in feet and hands) with oxygen therapy. At some point, studies may show benefit for oxygen therapy in not only relieving pain but also reducing symptoms. Borrelia and other intracellular microbes flourish in a low-oxygen environment. Forcing higher oxygen levels into tissues may create an unfavorable environment for these types of microbes.

SLEEP IS ESSENTIAL FOR RECOVERY

Beg, borrow, or steal—do whatever it takes to get a good night's sleep (with the exception of becoming habituated to a sleep medication); adequate sleep is essential for restoring normal immune function and overcoming CF/FMS. During acute flare-ups, sleep aids are often necessary to break out of the cycle of poor sleep. Start with natural substances, but sometimes prescription medications are indicated. Drug therapies, of course, should be limited to temporary and intermittent use only.

We'll work on your sleep habits later, but right now, let's just get you some sleep. When normal sleep is restored, the need for these supplements and/or medications will decrease.

NATURAL OPTIONS FOR SLEEP

Unlike natural supplement options for pain, natural supplements for sleep actually work fairly well. Many natural supplements have sedative properties that are useful for inducing sleep,[10] but a combination of bacopa, passionflower, and motherwort not only works well but also offers a very low potential for side effects and toxicity.

---

[10] Valerian root, kava-kava, and hops, commonly found in natural sleep products, are not recommended because of potential liver toxicity and potential problems with habituation.

- **Bacopa (Bacopa monnieri).** How about something that can clear your brain fog and also help you sleep? Bacopa is that something! Traditionally used in India for treating anxiety and insomnia, bacopa has been recently receiving much attention for improving cognitive function. Bacopa also offers adaptogenic properties for restoring balance in the face of stress.

  Dosage: 200–400 mg standardized to 50% bacosides at bedtime.

  Side effects: Enhanced cognitive function! (All side effects are not necessarily bad.)

- **Passionflower (Passiflora incarnata).** In its native Amazon, the woody vine of passionflower climbs into the rainforest canopy. When Spanish missionaries first noticed passionflower, they believed the large white flowers with pink centers resembled the crucifixion of Christ. Local inhabitants enjoy the fruit, but the medicine is actually derived from the leaves of the plant. Passionflower is now grown worldwide, and the beneficial properties of passionflower are well known.

  Offering both muscle-relaxing and sedative properties, passionflower has long been used for relieving nervous tension and restoring normal sleep. It has a reputation for restoring restful sleep without causing a next-day hangover.

  Dosage: 150–300 mg of 10:1 extract at bedtime.

  Side effects: Rare.

- **Motherwort (Leonurus cardiaca).** Traditionally used for relieving palpitations associated with menopause, PMS, and general nervousness, motherwort offers sedative properties and helps restore normal sleep. It has been noted to be particularly beneficial for 3 a.m. awakening. Though used primarily as a sedative, motherwort is strongly protective of nerve tissue and also protects mitochondria. It is a great supplement for restoring normal vascular function (normalizes blood pressure) and supports normal heart function. Motherwort has been noted to have antiviral and anticancer properties.

Dosage: 100–200 mg at bedtime (use higher doses of 400–500 mg if used alone).

Side effects: Rare.

A combination of bacopa, passionflower, and motherwort works well to induce and maintain normal sleep. Take the recommended dose of all three together before bedtime. Add a low dose of melatonin to initiate sleep and you have a functional sleep-management program—without the use of toxic and habituating drugs! The dose can be repeated once during the night if you wake up and cannot get back to sleep. Next-day hangover is unusual.

- **Melatonin.** Often used as a sleep aid, melatonin is primarily beneficial for inducing sleep, but less beneficial for maintaining sleep. It can be used in combination with the above supplements. It has potent antioxidant and neuroprotective properties.

  Dosage: Start with 1 mg. Sublingual (under the tongue) dosing is preferred because it more closely mimics natural melatonin secretion. The dose can be repeated with waking in the middle of the night to re-initiate sleep. Limit to a maximum dose of 5 mg over a 24-hour period.

  Side effects: Melatonin carries no risk of tolerance or dependence. Patients with significant depression should avoid melatonin.

PHARMACEUTICAL OPTIONS FOR SLEEP

- **Benzodiazepines.** These commonly prescribed drugs are very effective for treating insomnia and anxiety but are best used on a limited basis. Chronic use quickly leads to habituation and tolerance. They mimic the calming neurotransmitters in the brain but at the same time suppress these same neurotransmitters, which causes dependence on the drug. Some drugs work better for general anxiety (Valium, Klonopin, Xanax), and some work better for sleep (Restoril, Halcion). Acutely, these drugs work extremely well and are highly beneficial for occasional use. Chronic use, however, can turn into your worst nightmare!

- **Non-benzodiazepine sedative hypnotics (modern sleeping pills).** This relatively new class of drugs works similarly to benzodiazepines but is selective for inducing sleep. These drugs are very effective for inducing sleep but are highly habituating and come with the same problems as benzodiazepines. Ambien (zolpidem), Lunesta (eszopiclone), and Sonata (zaleplon) are the most common brands. Occasional use is okay, but chronic (nightly) use should be avoided.

- **Remeron.** An antidepressant with sedative characteristics, Remeron affects multiple receptors in the brain associated with sedation (as with most drugs, we don't know everything about how it works) but is less associated with adversely affecting the balance of normal calming neurotransmitters of the body. Remeron has less potential for habituation than other sedative hypnotics, and tolerance seems to occur more slowly. Remeron works well as an adjunct for treatment of insomnia. It is administered in small doses before bedtime (¼ to ½ of 15 mg tablet). The primary side effect is next-day sedation.

Now that you have adequate support for healing and we have addressed symptoms of pain and insomnia, it's time to start becoming proactive in your recovery. Time to put on your climbing shoes and make your way up and out!

PART THREE

GET YOUR FEET ON SOLID GROUND!

Supportive therapies can do wonders, but they will never alone get you up to solid ground. You must create an optimal environment for healing inside your body before you will move upward. Four major attachments are holding you down (processed food, toxic threats, perceived stress, and inactivity). Each of these sandbags must be released and allowed to fall to the bottom of the well before you will ever make it to the surface. The chapters in this section will help you let go!

We live in very unique times. Before 1940, people ate whatever they could get. Today in the developed world, people have a choice to eat whatever they want. And most of those wants are driven by primal urges for fat and starch and catered to by the processed food industry. Chapter 7, "Nourish," will free you from being a slave to food that comes only in a package.

These unique times are saturated with toxic threats of many varieties. Chapter 8, "Purify," will help you reduce your exposure to all toxic threats and free your body of toxic burdens.

We are all running from the tiger, every minute of every day. Humans seem to thrive on it, but it is another superficial attachment that can be modified. Chapter 9, "Balance," will show you how to put the tiger back in the cage (and keep it there). This chapter also covers thyroid dysfunction, hormone imbalances, and sleep.

Movement is essential for life. Inactivity, however, is more compatible with human nature. This is especially true with CF/FMS, where movement can actually be painful. Chapter 10, "Restore," offers advice for overcoming the natural tendency for inactivity and for restoring natural movement to your body.

CHAPTER 7

NOURISH

I magine biting into a piece of fruit, the sweet juice running down your chin and the mildly firm texture of the flesh unmistakably defining it as being a soft ripe pear. By purpose and design, the fruit nourishes seeds inside, but as a creation of life, the fruit of the pear also nourishes everything it comes in contact with. The energy contained in that pear can be referred to as vital energy—it is the energy that makes life possible.

All living things—plants and animals, and even bacteria—contain vital energy. When living plants and animals are harvested for food, the vital energy is transferred to the creature consuming the food, a necessary step in the circle of life. Defining vital energy in absolute terms is challenging, but most people intuitively know what it means. The definition goes beyond protein, carbohydrate, and fat found in food sources. It does include a spectrum of other nutrients necessary for life: water, antioxidants, vitamins, minerals, and, very importantly, enzymes that aid in digestion.

Vital energy does not stay around long, and fresh is always best. We do live in a time when fresh food is more available than ever before, but buying fresh food for every meal is not often practical. Fortunately, refrigeration prolongs vital energy in food, and freezing can extend it indefinitely. Canning works for some things, like beans, tomatoes, and oily fish, but the high heat used in canning reduces the nutrient value (and vital energy) of many other foods. Drying is a practical way to preserve vital energy in beans, whole grains, fruit, and certain vegetables, minus one vital component that can be restored—water. Drying is also useful for preserving the immense vital energy found in herbal medicines. Lastly, friendly bacteria found in fermented foods offer a whole different level of vital energy that is important to a healthful diet.

All food originates from living sources, but the vital energy contained in food is very dependent on how much the food source has been artificially manipulated. Use of artificial fertilizers and pesticides takes away vital energy. Industrial farming of single food sources decreases vital energy. Extensive manipulation by hybridization or genetic engineering (wheat, corn, and soybeans are the most affected) creates very unnatural foods deficient in vital energy. Processing food with machinery and packaging further degrades vital energy. Meat tainted by these unnatural food sources and produced under unhealthy (and some would say inhumane) conditions is robbed of vital energy. Regularly consuming these types of food robs vital energy from your body.

> To overcome CF/FMS, you must develop a new relationship with food. Food must be considered for how it will enrich your body with vital energy instead of how it will satisfy cravings. You must saturate your body with vital energy. Every morsel must be carefully scrutinized. This is very contrary to how your brain is programed to think about food. Your brain is programed to seek out sources of energy (carbohydrates, fat, and protein), but the programming was written long before processed food came on the scene. You must reprogram your brain to embrace natural foods providing intense levels of vital energy!

BASIC FOOD GUIDELINES

Make room for the good stuff!

To make room for all the wonderfully nutritious vital energy-enhanced food that can restore your body back to normal health, you must give up the processed food attachments that got you into this situation in the first place!

- **Time to give up food attachments.** You eat what you eat now because you are used to it and because the food industry has trained you and the rest of America to eat that way. If you had been raised in India or Asia, you would be comfortable with a whole different assortment of foods. Food attachments are really very superficial; they can be changed. It takes 60 days to break an old habit and form a new one.

- **Giving up wheat products is a good place to start.** Most people with chronic disease notice almost immediate improvement by simply avoiding products derived from modern wheat (white or whole grain, it really doesn't matter). Yes, it means giving up breads, cookies, cakes, cereals, and the like, and no, it does not mean substituting in gluten-free breads, cookies, crackers, cakes, cereals, and the like (they are made from processed rice starch, corn starch, tapioca starch, and/or potato starch and are just as bad). Other gluten grains (rye, spelt, kamut, barley) should also be avoided while recovering from chronic disease. While you're at it, you might as well give up the potato chips and cheese doodles. (Do you want to get well or not?)

- **Refined sugar (in any significant amount) and concentrated fruit sugar (fruit drinks) must be severely restricted while overcoming CF/FMS.** Gas-producing pathogens in your GI tract that feed off this stuff will be offended, but your normal flora will thank you by tomorrow!

- **Corn can also be a problem.** You can have corn on the cob in the summertime, organic corn chips with salsa, or occasional popcorn (I wouldn't think about taking those things away); it's the refined corn found in processed food products and drinks containing high-fructose corn syrup, corn oil, and/or corn starch that cause damage. These unnatural food products are not fit for human consumption (or animal consumption, for that matter). Soybeans, another source of refined oils and processed protein, are just as much of a problem.

- **The corn and soybean problem shows up in grocery store meat.** Nothing plumps up a chicken like corn. Have you seen the size of those chicken breasts at the grocery store? It can't be good for the chicken, or you. And visiting a modern pork-producing facility will definitely curb your appetite for pork. Corn fattens livestock faster than any other food source on the planet. Soybeans are thrown in the mix to add protein, but the meat is far from healthful. And with all the other additives, most grocery store meat becomes highly suspect. During recovery, this type of meat should be avoided completely.

- **Processed meat products (hot dogs, sausage, processed sandwich meats) should also be avoided completely.** If you take the time to research what they put in that stuff, you really won't want to eat it anyway.

- **Any kind of refined oil should be avoided.** All of your cell membranes will love you for it! Hydrogenated oils found in processed food products are especially harmful.

- **Deep-fried foods should never touch your mouth.** Frying food in hot oil creates fats that are completely foreign to the human body.

- **Almost all dairy products should be avoided during recovery from chronic disease.** The exception is plain yogurt or kefir and a limited amount of shredded cheese on top of salads or other foods. You'll be able to eat ice cream and cheese again one day, but let's hold off for a while.

Elevated insulin levels associated with insulin resistance and/or elevated blood glucose levels associated with pre-diabetes or diabetes are major system disruptors that must be addressed for recovery to move in a positive direction. The solution is, of course, strict control of processed carbohydrates. Metformin is a safe, well-tolerated drug that can expedite the process of restoring insulin levels to normal. It is one of the few drugs that truly supports the healing process. Self-monitoring with a glucometer from the pharmacy is a good practice in self-awareness (see Chapter 4, "Establishing a Baseline"). Hemoglobin A1c (target <5.3) and fasting insulin levels (target <10) are also important markers for defining these abnormal processes and monitoring improvement.

The body responds to living food.

We are truly living in the golden age of food—a privileged time when living food is more available than ever before. Living food is food close to its natural origins that has not been artificially manipulated. It provides antioxidants, enzymes to enhance digestion, and a host of vital nutrients! Embrace living food to restore vital energy to your life!

- **Ounce for ounce, vegetables contain more vital energy than any other food source.** Half of your food every day should come from fresh vegetables. This may sound like a tall order, but it's easier than you think. Varieties of vegetables mixed together and combined with other flavors and spices create wonderful taste sensations. Tastes of fat and sweet must be appeased, but this can be done in a healthful fashion. Coconut oil, avocados, and nuts are healthful sources of fat, and dried fruit or sweet vegetables such as tomatoes or onions can provide just the right amount of sweet to any food creation.

- **An apple a day, or blueberries...or cherries.** Berries and other temperate fruits are loaded with antioxidants and other disease-fighting substances. Melons provide glutathione and superoxide dismutase (which destroy free radicals) and a variety of antioxidants. Papaya and pineapple contain protein-digesting enzymes that are known to reduce inflammation. All natural fruits offer benefit, but because of the sugar found in fruit, daily vegetable consumption should out always outweigh fruit consumption.

  Think VEGETABLES and fruit.

Vegetables and fruit provide an excellent source of hydration. Because the water is trapped inside cells, it is slowly released during digestion, therefore adding water to the digestive process instead of taking away from it. Compare this to processed food products, which are nearly devoid of water. It's no surprise that it takes a 16 oz. drink just to get fast food down. But the liquid in the drink is quickly absorbed, leaving behind a dehydrated lump for the stomach and intestines to deal with—just another reason to give up processed food!

- **Beans are an excellent source of nutrition and vital energy.** High in protein and low in fat, beans contain complex carbohydrates that are slow to break down and do not raise blood glucose levels. Beans are also rich in flavonoids, substances with antioxidant power and the ability to balance hormones...and they really are good for your heart.

  The range in types of beans is broad. Mung beans (yes, there is such a thing; they do not need to be soaked, are quick to cook, and taste great!) and lentils are the easiest to digest of all beans. Red, black, and white...the variety of beans is almost endless. White kidney beans contain a substance that blocks breakdown of carbohydrate. Beans are healthful additions, whether used fresh, dried, or from a can.

- **Nuts provide healthful fats and many vital nutrients.** Pecans, walnuts, almonds, cashews, and other nuts should be considered healthful additions to your diet, but take note: Sensitivities to tree nuts and peanuts are common. If you have nut sensitivities, leave them off the list until your GI tract is healed. Also, peanuts grow a fungus that produces aflatoxins, a potent carcinogen—best leave them off the list completely. Sunflower seeds and pumpkin seeds offer nut alternatives that are well tolerated during recovery. Sunflower butter is a great substitute for peanut butter.

- **Whole grains can be healthful food sources.** Once artificially manipulated grains (wheat, corn) are excluded, other grains that can be enjoyed as part of a healthful diet include oats (gluten-free oats are available), brown rice, buckwheat, and quinoa. Eating the whole grain is preferable to using flour to create food products.

- **Eat enough, but not too much, protein.** Americans seem to be really hung up on getting enough protein. The daily protein requirement for normal health is about 60 grams per day. (A 3 oz. piece of lean meat provides 20 grams of protein; 1 cup of beans provides about 16 grams of protein; 8 oz. of yogurt provide about 11 grams of protein.) A little extra will not hurt you, but a diet heavy on protein is both acidifying and inflammatory. A high-protein diet will compromise your recovery.

  - ◆ **Fish/seafood is an excellent source of protein and the best source of omega-3 fatty acids.** Reasonable consumption is 3–4 times per week.

  - ◆ **Meat is a reasonable source of protein if the animals are fed natural foods and raised under humane conditions.** A good rule of thumb is poultry 1–3 times per week and beef or similar meats 1–3 times per month. Pork should probably be limited to 1–3 times per year (if eaten at all).

  - ◆ **Meat is not essential.** Farm-raised eggs, tofu, tempeh, and rice with beans are alternative protein sources that provide all of the essential amino acids. The seaweed spirulina is also a good complete protein source (add it into smoothies). Whey protein powder is also great for smoothies.

- **Healthful oils are oils that have not been refined with high heat or chemicals.** Cold-pressed olive oil and sesame oil are high in very favorable monounsaturated fats. Avocados and walnuts are a whole-food source of monounsaturated fats. Coconut oil contains medium-chain triglycerides that are very resistant to oxidation.

- **Vinegar is the most important vital energy condiment.** Vinegar is wonderful for adding flavor to food and is a primary component of many condiments, including mayonnaise, catsup, and salad dressing. It improves digestion and increases absorption of calcium.

- **Organic is generally worth the cost in terms of vital energy.** Food created naturally in the absence of artificial pesticides and fertilizers is the essence of real food. It is the ultimate way to boost your vital energy!

- **At least 70% of your food should be label-free.** Any food with a label on the outside is, technically, commercially processed food. Of course, it's impractical to make everything from scratch. The guiding principle for buying packaged, canned, or bottled products (catsup, mayonnaise, or hummus, for example) is whether you **could** have made that product at home from scratch with the ingredients listed on the container. Look for organic and fresh. Avoid products with ingredients with unfamiliar names or chemical additives. Of course, if you have time, anything made from scratch with fresh ingredients is better!

- **Life does require a bit of sweet from time to time.** Honey is a reasonable option for adding sweetness if used in small amounts. Refined sugar should be avoided. Stevia is the most acceptable sugar alternative because it is plant-derived (unlike other chemically formulated sugar substitutes). Some brands of stevia have better flavor than others.

The high cost of healthful food? You can actually buy a lot of good food for not much money if you stick to local produce, local eggs, and dried beans and cut back on your meat consumption (meat is really expensive). But even if you decide to invest more money in organic non-local foods such as fresh broccoli or blueberries shipped from another location, or organic meat fed natural foods, the cost will be deferred by spending less on medical bills and drugs later.

A healthy body requires adequate hydration.

Pure filtered water is the absolute best form of hydration for the body, but unless you are really thirsty, just plain water is pretty boring. Water that has been flavored in some way can be just as healthful (when natural sources are chosen) and is a lot more satisfying. There are many options for flavoring water.

- **Tea is possibly the oldest way to flavor water.** The tea plant originated in China but is now cultivated many places and enjoyed around the world. Green tea comes from fresh leaves that have been fermented and gently dried; all the important antioxidants and disease-fighting substances are retained. Black tea, more familiar to taste buds of those of European descent, is dried in the sun (oxidized), hence the dark beverage. White tea is made from delicate new leaves that have just budded. It may be the healthiest of all. White and green teas are lower in caffeine than black tea and coffee, and decaffeinated tea is an option if sleep disturbance is a concern.

- **Rooibos tea is the South African tea alternative.** Beyond being flavorful, naturally sweet and caffeine-free rooibos is packed with antioxidants and offers antiviral and anticancer properties. Rooibos is also known to alleviate constipation. It is an extremely good beverage choice for regular consumption during recovery from CF/FMS.

- **Herbal tea is another option.** Many herbs can be used to make flavorful teas. Different herbs can be combined for flavor or medicinal value.

- **Coffee should be mostly avoided during recovery.** Coffee is full of antioxidants but is also a gastric irritant. It can be resumed when gastrointestinal function is back in normal working order.

- **Citrus (lime, lemon, or orange) in water is a great option.** Sweeten with stevia.

- **Peeled cucumber in ice water provides a pleasant fresh, clean flavor to water.**

- **Whole strawberries in iced water provide a completely different taste sensation.**

- **Fresh herbs from the garden (dill, rosemary, or thyme, for example) are a great way to flavor water.**

- **Don't forget the water that comes inside fresh vegetables and fruit.** This can be a significant source of hydration.

Foods are important for reducing inflammation.

Certain foods increase inflammation in tissues. These same foods generate acid when they are metabolized. Other, more healthful, foods have the opposite effect and neutralize acid.

- The main inflammatory/acidifying foods include soft drinks, refined sugar, corn, wheat, oats, rice, dairy products, meat, refined oils, artificial sweeteners (especially aspartame), and alcohol drinks. High-protein diets are both acidifying and inflammatory. High-protein diets also increase risk of osteoporosis and kidney stones. Though some foods on the list can still be included as part of a healthful diet (oats, brown rice, and organic natural meat), they should always be balanced with alkalinizing foods.

- Anti-inflammatory foods also neutralize acids. Examples include all fruits and vegetables (just another reason to eat your vegetables!), pumpkin seeds, flax seeds, coconut oil, olive oil, sesame seeds, almonds, Brazil nuts, avocados, lima beans, white beans, lentils, tofu, Stevia, sea salt, and alkalinized water. Alkaline grains include buckwheat and quinoa.

Vinegar has the unique property of being acidic in the bottle but alkaline when absorbed into the body. When consumed, vinegar provides acetic acid that will enhance digestion in the stomach. Acetic acid is neutralized when food arrives in the small intestine, and acetate, a buffer, is then absorbed into the bloodstream. Once absorbed, acetate neutralizes acid in tissues.

TO COOK OR NOT TO COOK: FOOD PREPARATION

Food consumed raw preserves all the vital nutrients and energy but can also preserve some potential toxins and pathogenic microbes. Cooking prepares food for digestion, neutralizes toxins, kills pathogens, and makes certain foods taste better. Excessive heat from cooking, however, destroys nutrients and vital energy. The best answer is probably somewhere in between. Cook your food lightly and sometimes not at all. Some foods are best eaten raw, and others are better cooked.

- **Raw foods.** Uncooked vegetables and fruit provide high levels of vital nutrients and enzymes. Fruit is usually consumed raw, and most everyone knows the pleasure of a fresh mixed garden salad. It is possible, however, to follow an entirely raw-food diet. Raw-food diets are packed with vital energy and definitely support health restoration. Please note, however, that raw-food diets must comprise very fresh fruit and vegetables. Fruit in general and berries in particular grow toxin-producing fungus very rapidly. If all of your food is going to come from raw food sources, the food must be properly prepared to enhance digestion.

  If you are interested in the topic, there are many books written on raw-food diets. These publications will help you choose the right foods and teach you how to prepare them properly (which is really important if you want to gain the most value from a raw-foods diet).

- **Juicing.** Fresh juice from vegetables and fruit is very satisfying and healthful. Juicing, however, can be very expensive because a large amount of fruits and vegetables is required for a small amount of juice. In addition, all the fiber, which may be the most important part of the vegetables and fruits, is generally discarded. If you juice regularly, make sure you also include plenty of whole vegetables with other meals.

- **Churning/grinding.** Using a high-speed blender to churn vegetables and fruit together into a smoothie is a great way to prepare food. The grinding process breaks down fiber and releases nutrients but still retains the fiber; this allows easier digestion. Vegetable and fruit fiber is the best type of fiber for removing toxins, lowering cholesterol, and improving digestive function. There are machines designed specifically for this purpose (though a regular blender generally suffices), and plenty of recipes for smoothies on the Internet. Make sure, however, that the recipe is weighted more toward vegetables than fruit and that extra sugars are not added. Use honey or stevia if you need sweetness.

- **Steaming.** Light steaming may be the most healthful way of all to prepare food. Steaming breaks down fiber and releases nutrients, allowing easier digestion, without destroying vital nutrients. Steaming does not remove water from the food. Steaming (or any type of cooking) can destroy potential pathogens. Steaming works especially well for vegetables, seafood, and fish. Steaming is the absolute best way to prepare food while recovering from chronic disease.

- **Low-heat sauté.** Sautéing with low heat is very close to steaming (but more tasteful). Sautéing is a wonderful way to combine the flavors of a variety of vegetables and other foods (meat, seafood, and sometimes fruit) with herbs and spices. A wide, shallow sauté pan is placed over low to medium heat (never high heat!). A small amount of oil (olive, sesame, or coconut) is added, and onions, mushrooms, peppers, and meat (generally a small amount) are cooked first. The pan should never get hot enough to brown the food or burn the oils (gentle cooking). All the other ingredients are then added, including liquids such as soy sauce or vinegar and, if needed, vegetable broth. Temperature is reduced to low, and the pan is covered until all ingredients are tender but not overcooked. An endless variety of tasteful meals can be quickly prepared by this method.

- **Cooking under pressure.** As a quick way to prepare nutritious meals, pressure cooking seals in nutrients and moisture. The end result is very similar to steaming, but in less time and with less energy.

- **Boiling.** For most foods, boiling leaches nutrients from food and should be avoided. Eggs and shrimp are possibly the only reasonable applications of boiling to food.

- **Baking.** Casseroles and baked vegetables are flavorful dietary additions (and no one wants to miss out on Thanksgiving turkey), but baking does use lots of energy and tends to overcook food (which reduces vital nutrients).

- **Grilling.** Grilling is an excellent way to prepare meat of any type, especially if the food is not placed directly over the coals or burner and the grill is covered during cooking. This prevents charring and helps retain moisture in the meat. Vegetables can also be cooked inside a covered grill but should be placed in a container or foil to prevent burning and drying. Grilling does tend to dry food and does add minute amounts of unnecessary toxins; therefore, it should be reserved until you are well on the way to recovery.

- **Frying.** Using oil heated to a high temperature for cooking destroys nutrients and increases the fat content of food. The fats used in frying with high heat are altered and become free radicals. Frying food is extremely unhealthful and should be avoided entirely—always and forever!

- **Microwave.** Microwave radiation changes the chemical structure of fats and other chemical compounds in food; therefore microwave cooking should be avoided unless there are no other alternatives.

Breakfast smoothie: Toss blueberries, blackberries, ¼ banana, ½ peeled cucumber, spinach leaves, 1 scoop of whey protein powder, a splash of unsweetened coconut milk, and stevia to sweeten into the blender. Blend and then enjoy. A smoothie is great for getting down all those capsules!

THE "BEST" DIET

Note that healthful eating does not have to follow a particular doctrine or creed. The Paleo, Zone, South Beach, and other popular diets have made wonderful contributions toward better eating and dietary practices, but none are absolute. The most recent fad, Paleo diet, is restricted to foods eaten by humans in the pre-modern era. Although a true paleo diet is nearly impossible to follow (cultivated plants and domesticated animals did not exist 20,000 years ago), the modern-day version of Paleo is restricted to vegetables, certain fruits, and meat. The most healthful feature of the diet is exclusion of any processed foods. The diet, however, should not be used as an excuse to gorge on corn-fed meat (as some people do).

We can learn much about our food requirements from understanding human evolution, but it is not necessary to eat like primitive man to stay healthy. The best evidence of how we should eat comes from studying the diets of modern-day centenarians (people living to 100 years or beyond). Isolated populations of long-lived people exist around the world. In addition to long life, these groups also experience very low incidence of chronic disease.

The largest portion of their diet consists of fresh vegetables. They also eat beans and some whole grains (not allowed on Paleo). Meat is on their menu, but only from fish, seafood, and locally raised livestock—no corn-fed beef, and certainly no processed food. Other key factors to good health and long life demonstrated by these population studies include low stress, strong positive social ties, and frequent moderate exercise.[11]

---

[11] *The Blue Zones, 2nd edition,* Dan Buettner, National Geographic Society, 2012. *The Okinawa Program,* Willcox, Willcox, and Suzuki, Three Rivers Press/Random House, 2001.

MAKING THE TRANSITION TO HEALTHFUL EATING

When it comes to creating an optimal environment for healing, food is a great place to start. Set aside two weeks to embrace the concept of healthful food. Read through the food guidelines, and gradually replace foods that will impede your recovery with vital-energy foods. Take "Basic Food Guidelines" to the grocery with you and use it as a list. Create two areas in your pantry and refrigerator. Items that would be classified as acceptable according to the food guidelines are placed in one area, and everything else is placed in the other area. Gradually change the ratio until the "unacceptable" items are an insignificant part of the pantry and fridge.

Once your pantry and kitchen are saturated with vital-energy foods, the next step is transferring the vital energy into your body (and your family). Consuming vital-energy food is the exact opposite of boring. When varieties of healthful foods are combined with seasonings and spices, the results can be fantastic. It will not take long for you to realize how bland processed foods really are.

Recipes and inspiration can be found at vitalplan.com. If you need guidance on the basics of healthful cooking, I have a chapter on this in my first book, *The Vital Plan*.

NATURAL SUPPLEMENTS FOR NUTRITIONAL SUPPORT

The Basic Multivitamin

Vitamins and minerals should come mainly from a healthful diet, but a little insurance, especially while recovering from chronic disease, makes sense. When choosing a vitamin/mineral product, try to ensure that the vitamins and minerals should be presented to the body in the most natural form possible. Unfortunately, this important characteristic is not present in the vast majority of multivitamin products. Most multivitamins are made from inactive synthetic ingredients that are not readily usable by the body.

The best multivitamin products should state that the vitamins are provided in "active" forms and that minerals are organic chelates. The addition of herbal ingredients can be beneficial if the amount of each ingredient is stated. Products with long lists of herbal ingredients are generally not very valuable because the doses are too low. Products advertised as containing "whole foods" are generally not worth the cost—spend your money on real food. Avoid products with "proprietary blends," because you don't know what you're getting.

Omega-3 Fatty-Acid Supplement

The scientific evidence in favor of supplementing with essential fatty acids is hard to ignore. Essential fatty acids are important for decreasing inflammation in the body, supporting optimal cell membrane function, and improving brain function. The incidence of virtually all chronic diseases and some cancers is significantly reduced by the proper concentration of omega-3 fatty acids. A proper balance of omega-3 fatty acids is very important for CF/FMS recovery.

Though all types of essential fatty-acid supplements reduce inflammation, marine sources concentrate omega-3 fatty acids and work very well as supplements. Fish oils provide omega-3 fatty acids as triglycerides (pure fat). Freshness is the key to quality. A high-quality supplement should not have a "fishy" smell or taste. Another marine option is krill oil. The omega-3 fatty acids in krill occur as phospholipids, the natural form of the oil most easily used by the body. Krill oil is absorbed faster and easier than fish oil; therefore, "fishy taste" is less of a concern and less of the oil is required. Vegetable sources (e.g., evening primrose, borage oil, flaxseed oil) are also reasonable for supplements, but it generally takes a larger amount of the oils to achieve the same blood levels as marine sources.

When you reach a point that foods offering vital energy hold greater appeal than foods that simply satisfy cravings, you will have released one major attachment—one sandbag disappears into the depths below. Your load is lighter, and your body is now better prepared to gain upward momentum. But you are just getting started. Time to change gears and move on to the next major attachment!

CHAPTER 8

PURIFY

Life in the modern world is filled with invisible toxic threats that were not present a hundred years ago. Because these threats have not been around very long, humans really have little in the way of natural instincts to deal with them—you can see a saber-toothed cat coming from a mile away, but toxins in your food, water, and air may be just as deadly and are invisible. Buildup of toxins in tissues definitely inhibits healing and your ability to get better. You can't change the toxicity of the modern world, but you can learn to live around it. Doing this requires cultivating a new type of awareness.

Taking charge of the things within your control is the first step. You can control what you eat and drink. Certainly, anything applied to your skin is a matter of choice. Outside air quality where you live may be beyond your control (though you can make a plan to move if it's really bad), but the quality of air inside your home and workplace can certainly be modified. Possibly the most invisible and least controllable toxic threat we deal with is radiation, but reducing the threat is possible.

Enhancing the ability of your body to get rid of toxins is just as important as reducing the flow of toxins coming in. Although the body's capacity for removing toxins is expansive, the limits of detoxification are often surpassed, and toxins build up. Dietary fiber from all the vegetables, fruit, and beans (which you should now be in the habit of eating) pulls toxins from the body. Fresh vegetables and fruit also add water to support detoxification by continually hydrating the body; proper hydration is essential for detoxification.

A healthy liver is very important for optimal detoxification—take good care of it! Cruciferous vegetables, such as broccoli, enhance liver function and protect the liver. Normal kidney and intestinal function are necessary for toxin removal. Exercise increases blood flow and also causes sweating, both of which expedite removal of toxins from tissues. Many natural supplements protect liver function, improve bile flow, and support detoxification.

REDUCING THE BURDEN OF TOXINS

CURBING THE EVERYDAY THREATS

Toxic threats are subtly attached to things we do in life. Making minor adjustments in how you go about life is all that is required to release this attachment. If smoking and excessive alcohol consumption are not issues, then you are already two steps ahead. All you really have to do is become more conscious of where toxic threats come from and make a conscious effort to avoid them.

- **Strive for a goal of 75% organic food.** The most important foods to buy organic are thin-skinned vegetables and fruit: berries, apples, peaches, celery, peppers, spinach, lettuce, tomatoes, and potatoes, for example. Thick-skinned vegetables and fruit, such as citrus, melons, and avocados, generally do not have to be organic.[12]

- **Choose healthful meat.** Meat should be from animals raised humanely and fed natural food.[13] Wild-caught is preferred for fish and seafood. The cost is worth it; grocery-store meat is a source of hidden toxins.

- **Use filtered water.** Reverse-osmosis (RO) water filter systems are the most effective for removing toxins from tap water. RO filter systems can be purchased from any home-improvement store and easily installed within a couple of hours. The small investment is worth the peace of mind. If RO is not possible or available, use filtered bottled water.

---

[12] The Environmental Working Group (ewg.org) provides reasonable guidelines for food choices.

[13] EatWild (eatwild.com) provides lists of local farms producing better-quality meat products.

- **Breathe clean outdoor air when possible.** Breathing clean outdoor air is a matter of selecting a location known for clean air and of supporting clean-air legislation. If you live in an area where clean air is not guaranteed, be mindful of smog alerts and times of day when it is not a good idea to spend time outdoors. Also, get out of the city as frequently as possible and enjoy clean air.

- **Detox your home and workplace!** Most people spend more time indoors than outdoors, and high indoor air quality is easy to maintain.

  ♦ Change A/C filters regularly. Write a date on the filter so you know when it was placed.

  ♦ Self-contained free-standing HEPA air filters for individual rooms are very effective for cleaning indoor air.

  ♦ Replace indoor cleaning products with natural cleaners such as white vinegar and ammonia. Avoid using sprayed pesticides for crawling pests; use traps and solid baits instead.

- **Musty indoor odor signals a mold problem.** Mold and mildew are true health hazards. Mold growing inside dwellings, homes, and office buildings circulates toxins in the air that can compromise immune function. Symptoms of mold toxins vary depending on the immune status of the individual. Mold toxins are commonly associated with sinus and respiratory infections but can also cause chronic fatigue. Immune compromise leaves the door wide open for chronic infections with low-virulence pathogens.

  Moist environments such as bathrooms, kitchens, and laundry rooms often harbor mold, but mold can be embedded in walls and ceilings of any room in the house. Visible signs of mold are often hidden, but a stale musty smell gives mold and mildew away for sure. If the source of mold can be located and eliminated, that's great. If the odor cannot be easily controlled, however, call a professional and do whatever it takes to eradicate the mold problem.

♦ Consider placing a small dehumidifier in problem areas such as bathrooms to remove moisture.

♦ Clean moldy surfaces with chlorine-containing cleaners. (Chlorine is a toxin to you as well as mold; wear gloves and a chemical-filtering mask during application, and air the room until the chlorine smell is gone before using the room again.)

♦ Essential oils diffused into the air can help reduce the odor and mold spores present but generally will not eradicate the mold problem.

- **Quit smoking.** Use of tobacco products should be discontinued permanently; your recovery absolutely depends on it. It is impossible to smoke tobacco products and recover from CF/FMS. Try an electric cigarette. Get help if you need it (acupuncture, hypnosis, drugs), but you must stop!

- **Curb alcohol.** Alcohol is a toxin and should be avoided while recovering from any sort of chronic disease. Your body just can't handle any toxins right now. If you drink regularly, wean off slowly.

- **Be wary of exposing your skin to toxic chemicals.** If you must use toxic chemicals, wear gloves and a mask with a chemical filter.

- **Read labels on skin-care products.** Creams, lotions, and other topically applied substances are often overlooked as a source of toxins and allergens.[14] Seek out products derived from natural sources. Deodorant products not containing aluminum are preferred.

- **Use prescription drugs carefully.** Most prescription drugs are therapeutically dosed toxins. They are useful and important, but at the same time, drug toxicity must be respected. Most synthetic pharmaceuticals have direct toxic effects on tissues and contribute to decline in liver function.

---

[14] Environmental Working Group (ewg.org) regularly posts lists of safe skin-care products.

If prescription drug therapy is indicated, use the lowest dose possible to achieve the desired result. As your health improves, drug therapy can often be reduced or discontinued. Always talk to your healthcare provider about changing doses or stopping a drug.

PROTECTION FROM HIDDEN THREATS

In the modern world, we are constantly exposed to artificial electromagnetic radiation in the form of radio waves, microwaves, and radiation from electrical devices such as computers and cell phones. Eliminating exposure is impractical, but reducing exposure and gaining protection from this type of radiation is not only possible but smart.

- **Create distance.** If you can, avoid living near cell phone towers, radio towers, or large electric power grids; distance is the only way to limit this type of exposure.

- **Protect your vitals.** Laptops put out copious radiation. If you have ever experienced the "toasted legs" feeling that occurs while using a laptop, you know what I mean (more concerning are the vital parts also located in that general area). Fortunately, there are shields[15] available that, when placed under the laptop, block the majority of radiation. They actually work quite well. (I never use a laptop without one.)

- **Desktops computers are a little easier.** The processor can be located far enough away from your body not to be a problem. This is advisable, both at home and work. A shield can also be placed between you and the processor.

- **Be smart about your phone.** Cell phones are smaller than other types of computers, but are used often and are kept near or on the body continually. Shields can now also be purchased

---

[15] There are many different shields on the market, but the best one at this time is DefenderPad.

for cell phones, but how well they work is not well documented. Other ways to limit radiation exposure from cell phones include

♦ Using remote wireless headsets and car speaker/microphone kits whenever possible.

♦ Texting instead of talking (except while driving, of course).

♦ Not charging the cell phone directly beside the bed.

♦ Avoiding carrying a cell phone in a pocket with close contact to skin.

• **Supplement for safety.** Radiation causes damage that is very similar to that of free radicals. Antioxidant supplements can offer protection. Certain natural supplements have been defined by studies to offer protection from different types of radiation. Not surprisingly, many of the supplements discussed for essential support also offer protection against damage from radiation.

• **Review your radon risk.** If you live in a high-risk area for radon gas, have the crawl space of the home checked. Testing kits can be ordered over the Internet. A simple Internet search for "radon gas high risk areas" will tell you if there is need for concern where you live.

• **Use sun protection**. The sun is a potent force; spending a day in bright sunshine, even with sunscreen and protective clothing, can be quite debilitating. Clothing offers the best protection. Protection can also be gained from eating certain vegetables. Chemical compounds called carotenoids, found in yellow-orange vegetables, build up in the skin and retina of the eyes and counteract the damaging effects of sun exposure; two carrots a day is good for this. Lutein/zeaxanthin supplements offer additional protection.

Though using sunscreen is a good idea, many sunscreens contain chemical compounds that can become carcinogens when exposed to UV light.[16] Sunscreens block vitamin D synthesis. Limited sun exposure (20–30 minutes per day for several days a week) without protection is not harmful and is enough to generate daily requirements of Vitamin D. Even with sun exposure, having your vitamin D levels checked and supplement as indicated makes sense.

PRACTICAL PROTECTION FROM PATHOGENS

Toxins from CF/FMS-associated pathogens

Die-off of pathogenic bacteria such as Borrelia during treatment can cause significant symptoms. Pieces of the dead microbes (called endotoxins) are toxic to tissues and cause inflammation in small blood vessels. Endotoxins are typically very irritating to nerve tissue. Commonly called a Herxheimer reaction, the symptoms associated with treatment can sometimes be worse than the disease. Symptoms will gradually dissipate as therapy progresses, but there are things you can do to reduce the discomfort acutely.

- **Take sarsaparilla.** Sarsaparilla, one of the primary supplements discussed for Lyme disease, specifically binds endotoxins and can dramatically reduce Herxheimer symptoms. (Follow guidelines in Chapter 5, "Enhance Healing.")

- **Detox with chlorella.** Chlorella (see "Detoxify" at the end of this chapter) is a freshwater algae that binds toxins of many types and expedites removal from the body.

- **Get plenty of dietary fiber.** Fiber from vegetables and fruit helps pull all types of toxins from the body.

---

[16] The Environmental Working Group (ewg.org) regularly posts lists of sunscreens that are free of potentially harmful chemical compounds.

Reducing everyday exposure

Low-virulence microbes are always waiting to slip in through a crack in the doorway. They are the ultimate opportunists; don't leave your door cracked! A simple cold virus can suppress immune function, allow pathogens associated with CF/FMS to flourish, and dramatically slow your recovery.

- **Wash your hands.** Wash your hands or use hand sanitizers (these products contain only alcohol, which is toxic to microbes but not to you) after being in public and after exposure to other people.

- **Avoid heavily crowded public places as much as possible.**

- **Stay home when you are sick.** Please.

- **Take natural supplements.** Supplements with antimicrobial and immune-enhancing properties offer some protection against everyday viral illnesses.

- **Weigh the pros and cons of vaccinations.** Flu vaccines can protect you from coming down with the flu but can also cause flare-ups of chronic fatigue symptoms. Flu vaccines stimulate antibody production but, as a trade-off, may inhibit cellular immunity, allowing intracellular microbes to flourish. It's really a personal choice. In mild years, the flu vaccine may be best avoided; wait for the years when severe flu outbreaks with new viruses are predicted.

Taking the full regimen of supplements for CF/FMS may not prevent you from getting a cold or flu, but it can reduce the severity of the illness. The symptoms may also be atypical; instead of having typical cold or flu symptoms, you may only have exacerbation of chronic fatigue and related symptoms.

Cultivating healthy normal flora in your gut

If unnatural processed food has been your habit (notice the past tense; hopefully, you've seen the light by now), your gastrointestinal system is probably not functioning up to par. Processed foods compromise digestion, slow intestinal motility, and also encourage overgrowth of pathogenic microbes in the gut. "Bad bacteria" cause symptoms of gas, bloating, and abnormal bowel movements. These unfriendly bacteria can also produce toxins that have systemic effects. Buildup of bad bacteria can make you feel terrible.

- **Flush them out.** A common initial approach for dealing with toxic bacterial overgrowth is flushing the GI tract with a strong laxative. Functionally, this is what most "detox" products actually do. But you don't have to pay $20 for a laxative; a $1 bottle of magnesium citrate from the pharmacy will do the same thing. Once normal bacterial balance is restored, there is generally little need to repeat the process.

- **Don't feed them.** Eat enough nutrients and calories to supply your needs, but not enough to feed abnormal bacteria. Eliminating processed food will do wonders for eliminating bacterial overgrowth.

- **Take a probiotic daily.** Probiotic supplements (see "Detoxify!" in this chapter) reseed the intestines with friendly bacteria. They are very important for restoring normal gut flora.

- **Suppress their growth.** Many herbal therapies with antibiotic properties suppress "bad" bacteria in the gut but spare normal bacteria (another one of the great things about herbs over conventional antibiotics).

DETOXIFY!

Your body is continually detoxifying, but it always can use extra help. There's no magic here—if the amounts of toxins coming into the body are reduced and the body's ability to remove toxins is enhanced, gradually, the body will completely detoxify. There are four primary routes for removing toxins from the body: lungs (breathing removes CO_2 and certain other volatile toxins), liver-gastrointestinal (primary route of removal), kidneys (urine), and skin (sweating). Continuing good health habits will ensure that the body always stays ahead in the detoxification process.

- **You are what you eat!** Regular consumption of vegetables and fruit helps purge toxins from the body. Eating garlic and/or onions every day and artichoke whenever you can supports normal gut bacterial flora and enhances detoxification.

- **Keep well hydrated.** Clean, pure water helps flush toxins from the body. Do not overlook vegetables and fruit as another very important source of hydration. Vegetables and fruit are also alkalinizing, which aids in reducing risk of kidney stones and gallbladder stones. How much you drink each day is dependent on how much you sweat and how heavily you breathe during the day. The best guide is urine color: The color of lemonade is just the right amount, clear is excessive hydration, and the color of apple juice means not enough water.

- **Be kind to your liver.** Normal detoxification is very hard on the liver, especially in our toxin-saturated modern world. Certain vegetables, such as broccoli and other cruciferous vegetables, enhance the ability of the liver to neutralize toxins, especially estrogen-like toxins (xeno-estrogens). Many natural supplements are known to protect the liver. At the top of the list is milk thistle. Milk thistle improves bile flow and actually encourages regeneration of liver cells.

- **Exercise is essential for detoxification.** Exercise dilates blood vessels and increases blood flow. Improved circulation helps pull toxins from tissues. Exercise also induces sweating, another way to remove toxins from the body. Deep breathing improves lung capacity and increases removal of toxins through the lungs.

- **Address heavy metal concerns.** Historically, heavy metals have not been present on the surface of the planet to any significant degree, but industrial use in manufacturing and the burning of coal for energy have ensured exposure to virtually every living organism on earth. Unless exposure is excessive (occupational, dental fillings, smoking cigarettes), however, the body will gradually get rid of heavy metals (lead, mercury, cadmium). You can enhance this process by eating plenty of organic vegetables, exercising regularly, and breathing clean air. Because heavy metal toxins accumulate in fatty tissue, staying thin is not a bad idea.

- **Far infrared (FIR) sauna enhances removal of toxins.** This type of sauna uses radiated heat to induce sweating. It is possibly the most effective method (and safest) for removing heavy metals. Caution, however, is advised for CF/FMS patients because of the heat. If you chose to use FIR sauna, acclimate to the heat very slowly. Increase the heat in small increments with each session; stay plenty hydrated and gradually work up to higher levels of heat over weeks.

The best natural supplements for removing heavy metal toxins are alpha lipoic acid and glutathione. Chlorella and cilantro are often touted as good for removing heavy metals, but this is presently not supported by science. If exposure is excessive, FIR sauna may be the best (and safest) method of removing heavy metals.

NATURAL SUPPLEMENT SUPPORT

Liver support

- **Milk thistle (Silybum marianum).** Cumulative damage to the liver from a lifetime of neutralizing toxins is a significant factor in aging and disease. Silymarin, the primary chemical component of milk thistle, offers potent antioxidant protection for liver cells. It also increases natural antioxidants found in liver cells. Milk thistle has been found to induce regeneration of liver cells. It is the most widely researched of all hepatoprotective (liver-protective) herbs and is well known for low toxicity and high safety.

Suggested dosage: 400–600 mg extract standardized to 80% silymarin daily (1200 mg daily if liver enzymes are elevated).

Side effects: Very rare.

- **Andrographis.** This double-duty supplement with antimicrobial properties and liver benefit increases bile flow and protects liver cells (follow guidelines in Chapter 5, "Enhance Healing," for proper dosing).

- **Herbal support.** Most herbal supplements support normal liver function—just another distinct different between drugs and natural therapies.

Enhance removal of toxins

- **Chlorella.** Chlorella is a freshwater algae known for detoxifying properties. It is primarily effective for removal of organic toxins (but less so for heavy metals). Chlorella is also nutrient-dense, with high concentrations of vitamins, minerals, amino acids, and antioxidants. Chlorella contains many health-enhancing substances, but chlorophyll may be the most important for removing toxins.

Suggested dosage: Four (4) 500 mg tablets twice daily during detoxification. Look for pure organic broken-cell wall chlorella.

Side effects: None expected. Chlorella does contain iron. Men should monitor ferritin levels if chlorella is used regularly.

Enhance normal gastrointestinal function

- **Probiotics.** The "friendly" bacteria with best support from clinical studies include **lactobacillus** species and **bifidobacteria** species. Multiple species from these groups are generally found in most probiotic products.

  Suggested dosage: Bacterial concentration in products is defined by colony-forming units (cfu). For full therapeutic effect, 20–50 billion cfu per day are necessary.

  Side effects: Doses of up to 200 billion cfu are considered safe and are sometimes necessary for inflammatory conditions of the bowel.

- **Digestive enzymes.** Supplements containing enzymes to break down starches, sugars, proteins, and fat are essential any time gastrointestinal function is compromised. Most anyone over the age of 50 can benefit from an enzyme supplement.

  Suggested dosage: 2–4 capsules of digestive enzyme supplement with each meal.

  Side effects: Caution is advised if gastric or duodenal ulcers are suspected. (If burning occurs, discontinue use until healing of erosions is complete.)

- **Apple cider vinegar (ACV).** Apple cider vinegar improves digestion, decreases reflux, and increases gastric emptying. ACV also improves absorption of calcium. Take 2 tablespoons of ACV in 6 oz. of water with each meal. (Discontinue if severe burning occurs.)

- **Ginger and chamomile tea.** This flavorful tea is excellent for reducing inflammation in the intestinal tract. Chamomile comes in regular tea bags at the grocery. Grate about 1 teaspoon of raw ginger into a tea strainer and steep in a cup of hot water with the chamomile tea bag for several minutes. Sweeten with honey. Add a squeeze of lemon if you like. Take several times daily. Ginger is also an excellent antiviral.

- **Mild laxative.** Magnesium is probably the best mild laxative for use during detoxification. Milk of magnesia is the best choice for a mild laxative. Use only enough magnesium to allow normal daily bowel movements. Two teaspoonfuls twice daily is generally enough to provide a laxative effect. If chronic constipation is a problem, follow the advice of a healthcare provider.

SIMPLE TEN-DAY CLEANSE

The following simple protocol will decrease your exposure to toxins and enhance your ability to detoxify your body. Start the protocol on a weekend and continue it for 10 days. Allow several hours each weekend day to clean the house and change things around. The process requires a significant amount of physical activity and will certainly qualify as exercise.

Water

This is the easy one. Install an RO filter system to your drinking water supply. (Skip the single-canister filtering systems and filtering pitchers; they just don't do enough.) If an RO filter is not possible, start buying filtered water.

Air

If most of your time is spent indoors, this is where to concentrate your efforts.

- Thoroughly dust the entire house. Use a clean cloth and natural dusting solution. Mix ½ cup lemon juice with ¼ teaspoon lemon oil and ¼ teaspoon tea tree oil in a small spray bottle. A small amount will clean a lot.

- Invest in a good-quality bagless vacuum cleaner and vacuum the entire house. (If you have carpet in the main living area, clean it well. Whenever you change your situation, choose not to have carpet in the main living area!)

- Gather up and inspect all of the cleaning supplies in your home. Any products containing harsh chemicals should be disposed of properly. Replace them with natural products or cleaning solutions you make yourself. You can buy or recycle spray bottles. Vinegar, ammonia, and lemon juice/oil are great cleaning agents. Baking soda is useful when a little grit is required.

- Replace the filters in the air-conditioning/heat system.

- Purchase a HEPA air-filtering system and place it in your bedroom. The fan creates "white noise" that is great for sleeping!

- Repeat these steps at your workplace if possible.

Supplements

Enhance the detoxification process and restore normal gastrointestinal function by taking the supplements recommended for detoxification and restoration of digestive function. All supplements can be continued beyond the 10-day program.

Skin

Take stock of products applied to your skin. Products made from natural ingredients are generally better for your health.

Radiation

Use precautions for using electronic technology safely.

Food

The following dietary modifications will get you started on restoring normal gastrointestinal function, detoxifying, and eliminating food sensitivities.

- All processed food has to go—every single bit. This is a great opportunity to start cleaning out your pantry and refrigerator! Avoid all processed foods, all products made with any type of flour, dairy, red meat (beef, pork), and refined sugar as defined in the Chapter 7, "Nourish," guidelines.

- An optimal diet for detoxification should start with lots of lightly cooked noncruciferous[17] vegetables (squash, spinach, chard, carrots, celery, and the like). Onions, garlic, chicory, and artichoke promote growth of favorable bacteria in the intestines. Sweet potatoes are generally well tolerated, but regular potatoes should be avoided. Certain beans, including black beans, mung beans, and lentils are easy to digest and provide fiber for detoxification. Chicken, lean turkey breast, and whey protein are the best protein sources during the 10-day program. Non-oily fish are well tolerated by most people. Rice, oats, and millet are the best tolerated grains. (Rice and beans combined are a satisfactory protein source.)

- Wheat, nuts, yeast, tomatoes, citrus, eggs, bananas, beans, potatoes, soy products, pork, and beef are commonly associated with food sensitivities. Avoid them completely for the first 10 days. Then add them back, one at a time, and look for reactions of poor digestion or increased CF/FMS symptoms and pain for several days. If none occurs, that food (or food group) can be added back more frequently. Beef and especially pork, however, should be permanently placed on the occasional list.

- Seasonings and spices are not only allowed but encouraged.

- Steaming or low-heat sautéing with minimal oil is best for restoring function. Grilling should be avoided until GI health is restored; deep-fat frying should be avoided forever. Raw foods

---

[17] Cruciferous vegetables (cabbage, cauliflower, Brussels sprouts, broccoli) are very important for liver support and detoxification but cause gas and bloating in some individuals initially. If this occurs, avoid them until digestive function improves. (Digestive enzymes can help.)

should be avoided, except in smoothies (churning with a food processor or blender aids in the digestive process).

- Allowed beverages include herbals teas, green tea, white tea, and water with citrus (lemon, lime, orange) or other natural flavorings. Coffee and black teas are ideally avoided during the 10 days.

- You may eat ½ oz. of 60% dark chocolate if you need a special treat.

Sample menu items include:

- Breakfast: herbal tea and smoothie (1 carrot, 1 stalk of celery, spinach leaves, half an apple, ½ cup blueberries (or other berries), 1 scoop whey protein powder, ¼–½ teaspoon ginger powder, water or coconut milk, 1 tablespoon ground flax meal (optional).

- Lunch: steamed vegetables, rice and beans, chicken or fish, spices.

- Supper: sautéed vegetables, rice and beans, chicken or fish, spices. Use different vegetables, spices, and seasonings for variety.

- Snacks: carrots, celery, cucumbers with hummus, dates, apples, roasted pumpkin seeds and sunflower seeds with dried fruit, avocado slices.

- Salads with raw vegetables can be added back in after 10 days.

After detoxifying your body and infusing it with vital energy from healthful organic food, you should be looking skyward with a new positive attitude…but there is still more work to be done. Two more sandbags left. Putting that tiger back in the cage and balancing the hormones in your body come next!

CHAPTER 9

BALANCE

Modern life is stressful enough as it is, but having chronic fatigue takes escaping the tiger to a whole new level. Simple everyday responsibilities, such as having a job, maintaining a home, having a relationship with another person, or just dealing with life's red tape, can become major challenges. Add to that all the other things that inevitably pop up, and chronically stressed becomes a normal state.

Chronic stress affects everything. Your brain reacts to stress via your adrenal glands. The adrenal glands respond whether the stress is external (car wreck or boss yelling) or internal (the "I just can't take it anymore" kind of stress that twists your stomach into a knot and makes you want to throw up). You actually have two adrenal glands: one located on the top of each of your kidneys. The middle portion of each gland secretes the hormone epinephrine, better known as adrenaline. The outer portion of the adrenal gland secretes cortisol. These two "stress" hormones define how you will react to stress of any sort. With chronic stress, the adrenal glands become hyper-reactive and the stress response comes more quickly and is more intense.

Adrenaline is the hormone that prepares you for confrontation. Just the thought of conflict accelerates pulse, quickens reflexes, and sharpens mental function. The chances of survival in a real emergency are dramatically increased by the physiologic changes initiated by adrenaline. Survival is why we are here, and the adrenaline surge that keeps you in the game is actually quite invigorating. Our primitive man probably never felt more alive than when he had just escaped the jaws of a saber-toothed tiger. In fact, adrenaline is so intoxicating that humans tend to seek out conflict instead of avoiding it. It can all become overwhelming, however; the modern world is supersaturated with conflict. Too much adrenaline is disabling.

Cortisol is the hormone that directs the resources of the body to where they are needed for the given circumstances. When life is calm, cortisol secretion follows a gentle circadian rhythm that balances all functions in the body. During acute stress, increased cortisol secretion follows surges of adrenaline. Increased cortisol shifts the resources of the body away from everyday concerns (digesting food, repairing damage, normal immune functions) toward handling imminent conflict. The body is designed to handle conflict intermittently, but when the perception of threat never goes away, keeping the body poised in high alert 24/7 is quite destructive.

Ironically, the things you worry about most are not the real threats to your health. Real threats are mostly invisible (radiation, oxidative stress, poor diet, toxins, microbes). Things your brain perceives as threatening (marital stress, job stress, current world events, intense drama on television) threaten your health only by chronically increasing stress hormones. Sustained elevations in adrenaline and cortisol inhibit restful sleep, compromise digestive function, and suppress immune function. This strongly inhibits your ability to deal with the real threats. It becomes a vicious cycle that can result only in compromised health.

Adrenaline secretion is part of the autonomic nervous system, which regulates automatic functions in the body, such as heartbeat and breathing. Cortisol secretion is regulated by the hypothalamus, an almond-sized structure located at the base of the brain. The hypothalamus is responsible for regulating change, basically acting as the thermostat of the body. The hypothalamus is also the primary source of endorphins, the "feel-good" chemicals that control pain and boost immune function.

The hypothalamus exerts control indirectly by sending signals to the pituitary gland, which in turn regulates the adrenal glands, the thyroid gland, and the ovaries/testes. Together, they make up the central hormonal pathway of the body, called the hypothalamic-pituitary-adrenal axis, or HPA axis for short.

The autonomic nervous system and the HPA axis together control variations of normal functions in the body, including body temperature, thirst, hunger, weight, glucose, and fat metabolism; physical manifestations of mood; sleep; fatigue; night and day rhythms; blood pressure; heart rate; and gastrointestinal function. Everything that happens in the body is connected to these two pathways. Balance in HPA axis and autonomic nervous system is what good health is all about.

RESTORING BALANCE

Right now, adrenaline is not your friend. Chronic fatigue is like driving a car with a poorly tuned carburetor: Pushing on the gas pedal too vigorously will cause the motor to sputter and stall. For your body, adrenaline is your gas pedal. Push down on the pedal too hard (or consume caffeine), and your energy is going to sputter and fall precipitously. If you drive the car with a bad carburetor up a steep mountain, it's going to conk out about halfway up. It's the same with your body right now; you just can't tolerate stress of any kind—emotional or physical.

This is contrary to the way humans normally approach life. Adrenaline actually feels good. Humans thrive on stimulation and conflict (just pick up the paper or turn on the television). Life not pushed along by adrenaline is, well...boring. But this attachment to excessive stimulation must be suppressed for recovery to move forward. Time to take a big deep breath and say ohmmm-mmmmm...

- **Let up on the pedal.** Your approach to life needs to be calm and collected. This is a cultivated skill; it doesn't just happen. Note that the high points in life (being excited) can raise adrenaline just as much as the low points (feeling stressed out).

- **You have a stress threshold that precipitates symptoms.** Try to maintain stress below that threshold. As your health improves, you will be able to push down on the pedal a bit harder and enjoy a little more freedom.

- **Your world needs to be especially small (a primitive man's perspective, if you will).** If there is a tiger in the vicinity, you don't need to worry about it until it roars. A tiger on the other side of the world is the least of your concerns.

- **Shake off the little concerns and let someone else worry about them.** So many of the visible threats are not really threats at all. Let them go. Stop worrying about things you can do nothing about. Save your energy for the things that really matter.

- **Reduce unnecessary stimulation.** Turn off the news, and filter media. What's going on on the other side of the world or possibly even down the street is not your concern if it does not directly affect your well-being or help you achieve your goal. Pick movies, television shows, books, and other entertainment that enhance your motivation and raise your energy in a positive way. Don't waste time on media or entertainment that pulls you away from your goal of recovery.

- **Turn the volume down a notch.** Literally. Listen only to quiet, relaxing music for a change. Sometimes, pure quiet is best.

Entertainment with positive purpose can be good—an adventure when the good guy always comes out ahead, a fun comedy, a romance with a warm outcome, or a documentary that takes you to a special place. These forms of entertainment may raise your adrenaline, but they also stimulate endorphins and positive feelings. Entertainment with negative purpose—melodramas, horror films, or movies with bad outcomes—will raise adrenaline and cortisol. This type of entertainment can set you back for days, weeks, or even months.

Reduce the stress of everyday life. To overcome invisible threats that are the root of CF/FMS, you must reduce perceived threats and learn not to be driven or consumed by conflict.

- **Limit stress associated with work as much as possible.** Applying for complete disability is generally not necessary, but limiting the demands of work as much as possible should help your recovery. This may mean cutting back on certain luxuries and expenses, but it will pay off in the long run. The more time you can call your own, the better.

- **Call in favors.** You may have to rely on other people you can trust and cut back on your day-to-day obligations.

- **Avoid arguments you can't win.** Just walk away. Arguments raise your adrenaline levels and often waste your time. Pick your battles well—both at home and at work. This is a tough one, but you must learn to do it.

- **Make a pact with others close to you.** This includes spouses, children, friends, and coworkers—no arguments. Work out disagreements civilly.

- **Put your bills on cruise control.** Have monthly bills placed on direct withdrawal. Pay your daily expenses with a credit card. Stick to a budget. Absolutely do not spend more than you can pay off at the end of the month. Having to pay the bank interest on an overextended credit card is the worst type of financial sin. If you are already financially overextended, work with a financial manager and do whatever it takes to overcome the situation...and don't ever get into that situation again.

- **Try to limit travel as much as possible.** Travel is especially stressful for CF/FMS patients. Airline travel is especially stressful because of altitude changes, toxins in cabin air, noise, and exposure to microbes. When travel is a necessity, reduce the stress of travel as much as possible by planning ahead. Use of herbal adaptogens (see below) eases the stress associated with travel.

Protect your energy. Chronic fatigue is a state of low energy. Certain other people, situations, and places can deplete your energy levels. Recognize factors that drain your energy, and limit exposure to them as much as possible. Save up your energy before undertaking tasks or confronting people or situations that drain your energy.

- **Regularly seek out places or situations that renew your energy.** For some, these may be wide open spaces free of other people. For others, these may be quiet corners for meditation. Certain people may actually energize you; seek them out, but be careful not to drain their energy in the process. Upbeat music that you really like can also raise your energy level.

- **Negative energy drains your energy.** Avoid gossip and negative conversation. Suppress negative emotions.

- **Negative people will suck the life out of you.** Leave them behind.

- **Artificial sources of energy can scramble your energy.** These sources include computers, cell phones, large power transmission lines, and cell phone towers. Limit exposure as much as possible.

- **Raise your energy level with a positive attitude**. Try to look for the good in every situation and the bright side of every day. (This will also raise your endorphin levels.)

DEFUSING STRESS

Reducing the amount of stress in your life is a great strategy, but eliminating stress completely is impossible. You can, however, learn to defuse it. Like the gunfighter in an old western who faces his opponent while calm and collected with a steady gaze, you can manage even extreme stress. Staying calm in any situation is a skill that must be cultivated, but "calm like a gunfighter" is a really cool skill to have. All it takes is learning a few simple exercises. Regular practice of these exercises calms the adrenal gland and makes you more resistant to the negative effects of stress.

Assess tension.

How is your breathing? Quick and shallow breathing in the upper chest are signs of elevated adrenaline.

How cold are your hands and feet? Adrenaline causes constriction of peripheral blood vessels. A relaxed state is associated with warm feet and hands.

How tense are the muscles of the shoulders and neck? This is the first place that tension builds.

Diffuse muscle tension. One of the most obvious effects of built-up stress is muscle tension. Everyone tends to brace against pain, whether from walking outside on an extra-cold day or smarting from an injury; we reflexively tighten up the muscles of the back, neck, and shoulders and breathe rapidly and shallowly. Everyday stress causes the same kind of tension. Muscle tension increases pain. Learning how to recognize and release tension is essential for recovery.

Exercise #1: *Learn to recognize the feeling of your body bracing against stress. Every time you feel stress building, resist the urge to tighten up. Relax your abdomen and drop your shoulders. Loosen them up and let them fall until limp. Gently shake your whole body to release built-up tension. Lift your head and straighten your spine, like a string is pulling upward from the very top of your head. Your breathing will automatically slow down and become deeper.*

Relearn how to breathe. Breathing is your connection to automatic functions in the body. Being excited causes breaths to be quick and shallow. Excited breathing is associated with elevated adrenaline levels. Slowing the rate of breathing and breathing more deeply directly inhibits release of adrenaline. Heart rate decreases, blood pressure decreases, and systems normalize. This is how the gunfighter does it.

Exercise #2: *Observe your breathing while lying comfortably on your back. Control and slow your breathing to an easy rhythm. Place one hand on the abdomen, close to the belly button. As you breathe, try to keep the chest wall relatively still and pull air into the lungs by expanding the abdominal muscles. Your hand should rise and fall with each breath. Breathing should be done through the nose, not through the mouth. Ideally, inhalation (in-breath) and exhalation (out-breath) should be equal and the breath should never be held. It takes a little practice. Relaxation happens quickly, even after only a few minutes.*

Slow your breathing. The average person breathes about 12–15 times per minute when going about daily activities. An anxious individual may be breathing 30 times per minute—that's 1 second in, 1 second out. Wonderful things happen when you slow breathing down to 6 times per minute (5 seconds in and 5 seconds out).

Exercise #3: Using abdominal breathing, try to extend your breath for as long as possible without holding your breath. Inspiration and expiration should be equal. At first attempts, your inspiration and expiration will be about 5 seconds each, but your ultimate goal is to extend each to 15 seconds, resulting in only 2 complete breaths in one minute. Don't strain. Make it easy and comfortable. Work up to 15 seconds slowly. You can practice this anywhere, even at a stoplight.[18]

Slip into stillness. Periodically relaxing the brain reduces distractions and improves concentration. There are different levels of brain relaxation, with deep meditation being the most difficult to achieve. Mastering deep meditation, however, is not essential to achieve benefit. Simply reducing the flow of thoughts and relaxing the mind and body can do wonders. Your brain will be more focused, and life will be more enjoyable. Regular practice reduces adrenaline and cortisol, balances the HPA axis, and restores normal immune function.

Exercise #4: Find a comfortable position, sitting, standing, or lying down. Standing or sitting is preferred if you absolutely want to stay awake. Slow your breathing and breathe deeply into your abdomen. Imagine that you are sitting in an observation booth. A window allows you to see all of your thoughts, but you are not allowed to act

---

[18] A phone app called Insight Timer from spotlightsix.com makes this exercise really easy!

on them. Simply watch them float by. If a thought starts to gain trac-
tion, force yourself to let it go. Become a passive bystander. As time
passes, the frequency of thoughts will decrease and you will find your-
self gradually slipping into stillness.

Do a daily tune-up. Unlike your car, which needs a mechanic, your
body will tune itself...it just needs to be given the opportunity. A state
of low adrenaline, calm mind, and relaxed muscles is a perfect tune-
up environment. Just 20 minutes a couple of times a day will do the
job. The more consistent you are, the better you will feel, and this
may connect you to a side of life that you never knew existed.

Exercise #5: Lie down or sit comfortably in a chair. Slow your breathing
and relax your mind with the above exercises. Progressively relax your
body. Start at the top of your head. Become aware of the hollow spaces
inside your nose and ears. Become aware of your tongue and teeth. Spend
about 30 seconds or a few relaxed breaths at each location. Relax the mus-
cles of your neck. Become aware of the space inside your throat. Follow
breaths from your nose, down your throat, and into your lungs. Become
aware of your chest expanding and contracting with each breath.

Relax the muscles in your arms. Notice your heart beating. Move
expansion of breaths down into the abdomen. You may be able to
"feel" your liver and abdominal organs. Sit with a good posture, but
relax your abdominal muscles. Become aware of the pelvic area and
release any tension all the way through the anal area. Relax the thigh
muscles. Relax the lower leg muscles. Spread your toes, stretch your
feet, and then relax the foot muscles completely. Become aware of the
entire body all at once. Relax and turn healing over to your body.

Attitude is everything. A negative attitude can work against you
as much as a positive attitude can work for you. Have you ever
noticed when someone walks into a crowd beaming positive
energy with a smile, the whole room lights up? Both positive
energy and negative energy are powerful; it is up to you which
one you want to display. Displaying a positive attitude, even
when it is not the way you feel, raises energy levels, improves
confidence, and reflects to others that you have control over life.

SUPPORT WITH ADAPTOGENS

Hormonal imbalances (imbalances within the HPA axis) often respond well to adaptogens. Adaptogens are a special class of herbal substances known for balancing and restoring. All of the herbs defined as adaptogens have been used by humans for thousands of years and have an excellent safety profile. (Adaptogens were mentioned back in Chapter 5.) You may already be taking several (cordyceps, reishi, rhodiola, eleuthero). All adaptogens normalize immune function and balance the HPA axis, but each one independently offers slightly different benefit. Two adaptogens that are particularly useful for normalizing stress-related imbalances in the HPA axis include *ashwagandha* and *Panax ginseng*.

Adrenal overdrive

Prolonged emotional stress is commonly associated with high adrenaline states and elevated cortisol levels. Typically, a person suffering from prolonged emotional stress is fatigued, sleeps poorly, is overly anxious, and tolerates stress very poorly—basically burning both ends of the candle at once. High blood pressure and elevated pulse are commonly associated with this situation.

This type of adrenal dysfunction responds best to calming adaptogens such as ashwagandha, but other adaptogens mentioned in Chapter 5 can also provide benefit. Ashwagandha is especially beneficial for balancing the HPA axis. When combined with l-theanine, magnolia, and philodendron herbs, the effect can be remarkable.[19]

- **Ashwagandha (Withania somnifera).** Say it with a big voice, like you are reciting an incantation: **Ash-wa-GAND-ha!** The magic that it offers is real! Ashwagandha is one of the best herbs for balancing hormones and reducing the detrimental

---

[19] Patented-grade extracts offer the highest level of purity and efficacy. The product HPA Balance is a combination of three patented-grade extracts, including a patented form of ashwagandha called Sensoril®. This product has shown exceptional benefit for menopausal symptoms, stress-related conditions, and any condition associated with imbalance in the HPA axis.

effects of stress. Native to India, ashwagandha is revered for its ability to balance, energize, rejuvenate, and revitalize. Ashwagandha has been used for thousands of years as one of Ayurvedic medicine's (the traditional medicine of India) most revered revitalizers.

Ashwagandha is particularly useful for balancing the HPA axis. By restoring balance in this important pathway, ashwagandha improves stress resistance, allows for improved sleep, reduces brain fog and fatigue, and improves menopausal symptoms (especially hot flashes). These properties also lend to usefulness for controlling carbohydrate craving and weight loss. Ashwagandha also offers anti-inflammatory, antioxidant, anti-cancer, and immune-enhancing properties. In addition, ashwagandha is known to help restore normal thyroid function.

Suggested dosage: 200–500 mg of standardized extract twice daily. (Dosages vary per type of extract—Sensoril, a patented-grade extract, offers the highest efficacy.)

Side effects: Uncommon and mild. Ashwagandha contains iron and should be avoided by individuals with hemochromatosis (defined by high iron ferritin levels). Though ashwagandha is generally sedating, some individuals may experience mild stimulation.

Adrenal burnout (adrenal fatigue)

If intense stress is chronic—not just an occasional crappy day, but weeks or months of crappy days—adrenal "burnout" can occur, resulting in low cortisol levels. The body continues to be driven by high adrenaline release, but cortisol secretion starts to wane and the body can no longer keep up. Total collapse is the inevitable consequence. A person with low cortisol levels has absolutely no energy and sleeps excessively. This person goes to bed tired and wakes up tired. Sleep does not improve fatigue. Commonly associated symptoms include low blood pressure, low pulse, and depression.

This situation responds best to stimulating adaptogens such as Panax ginseng. Licorice is also well known for restoring adrenal function and normalizing blood pressure. Panax ginseng is especially beneficial when fatigue is associated with excessive sleepiness. In this case, guarana and yerba mate can provide added benefit and act synergistically with Panax ginseng. (All of these herbs are stimulating and should be avoided by individuals with high blood pressure, insomnia, or anxiety.)

- **Panax ginseng.** Ginseng supports normal adrenal function and improves energy levels. It may also improve mental alertness, concentration, and stamina. Ginseng is one of the most studied herbal substances in use. It is excellent for restoring normal adrenal function and balancing the HPA axis.

  Suggested dosage: 300–500 mg of extract standardized to contain 4%–7% ginsenosides 1–2 times daily.

  Side effects: Stimulation. Ginseng should be avoided in individuals with hypertension, heart disease, insomnia, or anxiety.

- **Licorice (Glycyrrhiza glabra).** Licorice is an excellent herb for restoring and supporting adrenal function. It will restore normal blood pressure and normal cortisol rhythms. Licorice also offers potent antiviral properties and immune restoration. Licorice is a great synergist with other herbs. It should always be used in combination with other herbs and never alone.

  Suggested dosage: 1–2 500 mg capsules (standardized to 24% glycyrrhizic acids) up to three times daily. Use should be limited to short duration, and recommended doses should not be exceeded.

  Side effects: Elevated blood pressure. Stimulation. Excessive or prolonged use can result in sodium retention and potassium loss, with high blood pressure and swelling.

OTHER HPA AXIS CONDITIONS

Thyroid dysfunction

The thyroid gland controls metabolism in the body. The hypothalamus, via the pituitary gland, controls secretion of thyroid hormones. This connection makes thyroid function part of the HPA axis. Virtually everything that happens in the body is tied to the HPA axis, so balancing the HPA axis is extremely important for normal health and recovery from disease.

Hypothyroidism (low thyroid) is the most common form of thyroid disease. It is a complex disorder, and dysfunction can occur in a variety of ways. The gland can basically "burn out" from exposure to stress factors. Also, antibodies (autoimmune) can damage the gland or block thyroid hormone from working. Iodine is necessary for the formation of thyroid hormones, and low iodine can lead to low thyroid hormone production and formation of goiter. Cysts and even cancer can form in the thyroid gland, compromising function.

Hypothyroidism is more common in women than in men, and some hereditary tendencies run in families. Associations have been made with wheat consumption and insulin resistance. Certain foods, known as goitrogens, can cause increased risk of hypothyroidism[20] when frequently consumed raw. Many toxins, including fluoride, chlorine, mercury, dioxins, and insecticides, have been implicated as causative in thyroid disease. Toxins and the rise in nuclear radiation may be contributing to the steady rise in thyroid disease occurring over the past century. Stress is definitely a factor. Trauma to the neck and chest can initiate thyroid disease. A link with microbes, both viruses and bacteria, is certainly possible.[21]

---

[20] Common goitrogens include cruciferous vegetables, carrots, corn, peanuts, and walnuts.

[21] Mary J. Shomon has written several must-read books about thyroid disease (see references).

Hypothyroidism is a function of the same system disruptors as CF/FMS. Not surprisingly, the two disorders share many, if not most, of the same symptoms. In fact, hypothyroidism could be considered just a variant of CF/FMS. In other words, most of the symptoms of hypothyroidism are caused by system disruptors affecting the entire biochemistry of the body and not necessarily by abnormal thyroid hormones alone. If the thyroid gland has been damaged, thyroid hormone replacement may be necessary, but if thyroid hormone replacement is the only therapy, many patients continue to be symptomatic.

Possibly the most important factor in treating thyroid disease is finding a provider who understands the necessity of treating the patient rather than just treating the numbers. Your primary care provider can manage uncomplicated thyroid dysfunction, but complex disease should be managed by an endocrinologist (a specialist in hormonal diseases). If you are diagnosed with hypothyroidism, your healthcare provider may discuss the following options for therapy.

Prescription medications for hypothyroidism

- **Levothyroxine** (Synthroid, Levoxyl, Tirosint[22]). The most commonly used standard for treating hypothyroidism is levothyroxine. Though synthetically derived, levothyroxine is bio-identical human T_4, the most abundant thyroid hormone in the body. Most people do very well with this form of thyroid replacement, but some people do not convert T_4 into the active thyroid hormone, T_3. These individuals tend to do better with natural porcine thyroid hormone.

- **Natural porcine thyroid** (Armour Thyroid, Nature-Throid). This natural product is derived from the thyroid glands of pigs. The fact that it contains all forms of thyroid hormone in

---

[22] Tirosint is a brand of levothyroxine that uses a hypoallergenic tablet. This is the best brand name to use for individuals with sensitivities to tablet fillers.

proper ratios provides an advantage for some patients. Porcine thyroid, however, is not bio-identical for humans. With time, some people will develop antibodies to the porcine hormone and the medication will lose its effectiveness. Note that dosing of different thyroid medications is not equivalent—100 mcg of levothyroxine is equal to 60–65 mg of porcine thyroid.

- **Human T_3 (Cytomel).** Human T_3 is a good option for select patients. It is usually combined with levothyroxine to mimic normal balance of thyroid hormone secretion.

Natural supplements supporting thyroid function

- **Iodine supplements.** Iodine supplementation is a controversial topic. Too little (about 20% of Americans are considered deficient) can lead to goiter and hypothyroidism, but too much can actually aggravate thyroid disease. The current recommended daily allowance (RDA) is 150 mcg per day, but many experts recommend more, especially if you do not use iodinated salt. Sea vegetables (seaweed) are commonly recommended as a natural iodine source, and it is true that sea vegetables offer the most bioavailable form of iodine, but the iodine content is highly variable between different sources. If you decide to supplement with more than the RDA, you may want to ask your healthcare provider about testing iodine levels,[23] especially if you have active thyroid disease.

- **L-tyrosine.** Thyroid hormone is made from iodine molecules attached to the amino acid l-tyrosine. Supplements can help support normal thyroid function.

- **Ashwagandha**. This previously discussed adaptogenic herb also stimulates thyroid activity.

---

[23] Urinary iodine clearance test.

Menopause

Menopause is a natural process; it is not a disease and is not directly caused by poor health habits. The natural midlife cessation of ovarian function signals the onset of menopause. Natural or not, however, the fluctuations in female hormones associated with menopause do cause significant disruptions of the HPA axis and autonomic functions. Body thermostat variations including hot flashes and night sweats, sleep disturbances, fat distribution changes, heart rate changes, and certainly fatigue are related to the abnormal feedback from the ovaries to the hypothalamus. Perimenopause, the stage leading up to menopause, includes all the above symptoms but can also include irregular and heavy periods. Symptoms are increased in women who follow poor health habits.

Usually, the best approach to menopause is a comprehensive approach. Women who follow good health practices generally have an easier transition through menopause. Herbal therapies that balance the HPA axis often relieve many of the symptoms associated with menopause. Natural progesterone cream applied to the skin daily (available over the counter) opposes estrogen dominance and helps prevent heavy periods during perimenopause. Natural progesterone also reduces menopausal symptoms and slows bone loss. The herb Vitex agnus-castus (chaste tree berry) is excellent for normalizing periods during perimenopause. After menopause, bio-identical transdermal estrogen replacement (with progesterone) properly administered in small doses can be life-altering.

Andropause

Decline in testicular function is common in men as they age, but, unlike menopause, decline in male hormone production is not a natural process and can be sourced to the factors that cause disease and aging. Hormonally active toxins, insulin resistance caused by excessive carbohydrate consumption, and stress are at the top of the list. Reduction of these factors can often normalize hormone secretion. Though testosterone replacement is becoming a common solution, giving testosterone hormone actually suppresses normal testosterone secretion and causes testicular atrophy (the gonads shrivel up). It has also been associated with increased cardiovascular risk. Dietary and lifestyle modifications are the most effective solutions. Herbal therapies can also provide benefit. Fenugreek, tongkat ali, and epimedium are a few examples of herbs that naturally enhance testosterone production.

Growth hormone

Growth hormone is another hormone that is often targeted for replacement in fatigue syndromes. Secreted by the pituitary gland, growth hormone has anabolic (building-up) functions in the body. Anti-aging practitioners maintain that because growth hormone declines with age, replacing growth hormone will slow the processes of aging—and it does...at least for a while. Replacement, however, suppresses natural growth hormone secretion, and the patient ends up being worse off in the long run. Also, growth hormone replacement is extremely expensive. A better strategy is supporting normal glandular function with good health habits.

There are small populations of people existing around the world who naturally enjoy extreme longevity and low incidence of chronic disease. Good health practices (low exposure to toxins, very limited use of processed foods, high intake of foods with antioxidants and vital nutrients, frequent moderate exercise, low stress, and intake of herbs with antimicrobial properties) are common to all of these groups. In groups where growth hormone was measured, it was found to be the same level as in much younger individuals.[24]

A GOOD NIGHT'S SLEEP

It's a simple fact: Recovering from CF/FMS is nearly impossible without good sleep. Sleep is the time when your body is in optimal recovery mode. Without sleep, all systems of the body suffer and the incidence of all diseases increases.

---

[24] *The Blue Zones, 2nd edition,* Dan Buettner, National Geographic Society, 2012. *The Okinawa Program,* Willcox, Willcox, and Suzuki, Three Rivers Press/Random House, 2001.

Ironically, however, poor sleep is almost always associated with chronic fatigue. It's really not fair. Normal people get sleepy when they get tired, but people with chronic fatigue typically get more tired and agitated at the same time. Sleep comes *less* easily. Chronic stress increases cortisol, and elevated cortisol keeps the brain alert. This, coupled with other factors, compromises sleep, especially deep, restorative sleep. It's just another reason to work hard at keeping adrenaline and cortisol levels at a low baseline.

The other factors adversely affecting sleep include pain, hormonal imbalances, inflammation, toxins, endotoxins from dying pathogens, and imbalances in gut flora. As these factors are reduced, healing occurs and sleep will gradually return to normal. You are not permanently broken—you will be able to sleep normally again. Sometimes, proper diagnosis involves a trip to a sleep clinic, such as with disorders like sleep apnea, restless legs syndrome, or narcolepsy, but for the garden-variety sleeplessness that occurs with CF/FMS, treatment is a matter of normalizing a hyper-stimulated nervous system.

PREREQUISITES FOR NORMAL SLEEP

- **Maintain low adrenaline levels during the day.** This is the key to restful sleep. Become a master of the simple breathing and focus exercises discussed earlier in this chapter.

- **Absolutely avoid caffeine** until sleep cycles return to normal. Insomnia will not resolve until caffeine is discontinued! Most beverages are available in caffeine-free versions. Look for hidden stimulants in supplements and foods. Be aware that many, if not most, medications disrupt normal sleep.

- **Avoid alcoholic beverages in the evening.** Alcohol initially is a sedative, but the metabolites are stimulants. Expect to be wide-eyed and awake about 3 to 4 hours after you consume alcohol. (It's best to avoid alcohol completely until you are well.)

- **Avoid commercially processed food.** Chemicals present in food products can irritate the brain and contribute to insomnia.

Hormonal imbalances associated with carbohydrate consumption may contribute to insomnia.

- **Be aware of toxins.** Certain toxins may irritate nerve tissue or have stimulating effects.

- **Sleep on a comfortable mattress.** Memory foam mattresses are especially conducive to a good night's sleep and allow sleeping on the side. Sleeping on one's back encourages sleep apnea.

- **Limit noise pollution such as snoring bed partners or restless pets.** Consider obtaining an electronic device that produces white noise to drown out surrounding sounds. Be aware that your bed partner may be keeping you awake. Movement and snoring from a person in the room may be contributing to insomnia. Consider sleeping in an isolated location until sleep is improved.

- **Avoid vigorous exercise after 8 p.m.** The exception to the rule is relaxing yoga routines. Exercise during the day, however, is excellent therapy for insomnia.

- **Take a brief "power nap" midday to calm the mind and body.** This allows for better sleep at night. Try to take a nap or at least turn your brain off at least once in the middle of every day!

- **Address chronic pain and chronic digestive disorders.**

- **Address menopausal issues.**

- **Try acupuncture and/or hypnosis.**

- **Get a sleep test.** If excessive snoring or the possibility of sleep apnea exists, visit a sleep clinic for an overnight stay.

- **Let your healthcare provider know if restless legs are a problem**. Generally, restless legs improve with improved health habits, but therapies are available that may help in the short term.

Out of desperation, many patients with insomnia turn to pharmaceuticals for relief. Although this would seem like a legitimate course of action, sleep-inducing medications can actually worsen the problem. As discussed in Chapter 6, sleep medications adversely affect the normal calming neurotransmitters in the brain. Habituation and dependence on these drugs is not where you want to go. If you are already dependent on a benzodiazepine or modern sleep medication, I encourage you to read The Ashton Manual (benzo.org.uk) and find a provider who can help you wean off gradually without compromising your recovery.

QUEST FOR A GOOD NIGHT'S SLEEP

- **Allow plenty of time for good sleep.** You may have to allow 9–10 hours each night to get 7–8 hours of quality sleep. Getting to sleep initially may take more time than for average people and getting back to sleep after early morning awakening will also take time. (It is very important that you try to get back to sleep; this is sometimes the most restful sleep of the night.)

- **Be very particular about your bedtime routine.** Try to set a pattern of going to bed and getting up at the same time each day. If you work a regular job, try to get into bed by 10 p.m. each evening. Respect normal day and night cycles as much as possible; let the sun dictate your sleep cycles.

- **Avoid excessive light stimulation in the evening.** Use low lights and turn off televisions and especially computer screens after 8 p.m. This will help stimulate natural melatonin levels. Try reading before bedtime, or try practicing relaxation techniques.

- **Always sleep in a very dark room.** Use heavy shades if necessary. This is especially important if you work night shift and sleep during the day.

- **Adjust the thermostat.** Being overly hot or overly cool can adversely affect sleep.

- **A calm day is the best recipe for a restful night.** Regular practice of relaxation techniques throughout the day makes for an easier transition into sleep during the night.

- **Establish a routine for falling asleep.** Take 10 minutes to progressively relax the muscles of the body.

- **Sometimes, a warm bath can help.** Being immersed in warm water can be especially beneficial if the body is tense and agitated.

- **Melatonin, 1 mg, under the tongue is often effective for initiating sleep.** This small dose can be repeated several times during the night with reawakening. Other supplements from the list below can be helpful.

- **If you become awake, don't cut the lights on!** Many sleep experts recommend that upon waking in the middle of the night, you should get up, turn on the light, and read or do some other type of activity until you become sleepy. Although this may work for some people, turning on the lights suppresses natural melatonin—this is the last thing you want to do! Instead, keep the lights off, have your MP3 player ready by the bedside, and start practicing relaxation techniques before the stream of verbal thoughts starts pouring in. Not only will you have made good use of valuable practice time, you will probably be asleep again before you know it!

Get pillow speakers! Yes, pillow speakers. They can be obtained through Internet sources. You can place them inside your pillowcase, and plug them into an mp3 player such as an iPod. Also order the Delta Sleep System (or similar audio program) as an audio download or CD. The Delta System is nonrhythmic music with delta waves (deep-sleep waves) transposed in the music that help induce the brain into sleep. Set the mp3 player on a continuous loop so the music plays all night. It actually works!

NATURAL THERAPY FOR SLEEP ENHANCEMENT

Best and safest options for sleep aids

- Combinations of supplements may not be quite as potent as pharmaceuticals, but they can be safely used continually. For a starting point, many individuals are able to control mild to moderate insomnia with natural supplements such as ashwagandha that balance the HPA axis.

- At bedtime, ½ to 1 mg of sublingual (taken under the tongue) melatonin is often effective for initiating sleep. This low dose of melatonin can be repeated several times during the night (up to 5 mg total) upon waking. Note that melatonin is a sleep initiator, not a sleep sustainer. Oral melatonin and time-released melatonin do not mimic the normal secretion of melatonin in the body and should be avoided!

- Bacopa, passionflower, and motherwort form a very useful and safe combination for restoring sleep. (See discussion and dosages in Chapter 6, "Symptom Control: Pain and Sleep.") This combination can be used safely until a normal calm state is established and normal sleep returns.

Supportive supplements for sleep

- **Lavender essential oil.** Put a few drops on your pillow to enhance normal sleep.

- **Chamomile tea.** Chamomile works great for some people but causes stimulation in others. Look for a bedtime tea blend that contains lemon balm and other sedative herbs.

- **Magnesium.** Magnesium provides an overall calming effect and relaxes muscles. Response to magnesium increases with dosage, but dosage is limited by gastrointestinal symptoms, predominantly loose stools. The average therapeutic dose is 400 mg of magnesium citrate or magnesium glycinate taken a couple of hours before bedtime. Magnesium glycinate is the most well absorbed form of magnesium and is associated with the least incidence of loose stools. Glycinate is also calming.

- **SAMe.** In addition to having anti-inflammatory properties, SAMe improves mood and helps maintain normal sleep. SAMe is also a mood elevator in individuals with depression. The incidence of side effects is low. SAMe should be avoided if taking antidepressant medications. The average dose for achieving beneficial effect is 600–1200 mg daily (making SAMe the most expensive choice).

Three down and only one to go…but letting go of stress was a big one! You should now feel stronger, lighter, leaner, and ready for the last challenge! Time to breathe life back into your body and start moving again!

CHAPTER 10

RESTORE

The most appropriate maneuver for escaping a tiger is running, but primitive humans did not actually spend much time running from tigers; encountering tigers in the primitive world was relatively rare. In actuality, moving as little as possible is more consistent with human nature. Movement requires effort and initially causes pain (and even mild exertion can cause discomfort for people with CF/FMS). Even so, life necessitates movement, and being active is essential for normal health. Pushing through the pain to get the gain is essential. Regular movement clears toxins from the body and generates endorphins. Being active is necessary for overcoming chronic fatigue. Inactivity is the last major attachment to release before you can reach solid ground.

Possibly the most healthful exercise is consistent with that of primitive humans. Primitive people did not do what they wanted to but what they had to do...and the main "had to" was collecting food. This required walking...lots of walking. In addition to walking, they had to stop and pick things up fairly frequently. Playing golf, walking the beach to collect shells, and picking berries in the woods are possibly some of the most natural forms of exercise. (Remember to protect yourself from insect bites!) Kayaking, rowing, biking, and hiking up and down small hills are pretty good too. Lifting heavy stuff occasionally and running short distances is okay (after you are warmed up), but bulking up is not (your ancient ancestors were lean bipeds, not Neanderthals).

Strictly from a health point of view (and not from an athletic point of view), moderate consistent movement is superior to brief episodes of intense strenuous exercise. This definitely applies to individuals with chronic fatigue. Regular exercise is very important, but intense workouts are not. In fact, they will work against your recovery. Consistent (daily, for as much time as you can spare) low-intensity physical activity is one of the best things that you can do to encourage recovery. It needs to be enough to raise heart rate, move blood around, and generate sweat. In addition to walking, yoga, Qigong, and tai chi are great movement exercises for CF/FMS!

> The longer you exercise, the more good you do. It takes about twenty minutes to warm up (this is the uncomfortable part). After the body is warmed up, wonderful things happen. Blood vessels dilate, and blood flow increases to all parts of the body. This removes toxins, lowers blood glucose levels, normalizes hormone levels, balances the HPA axis, and increases natural endorphins. (Endorphins are the "feel-good" chemicals that boost immune function.) Thanks to endorphins, exercise is one of the best antidepressants around. Again, it doesn't take intense exercise to gain all the benefits, only consistency! The more you do it, the better you will feel!

RECOVERY IN MOTION

Your body is your vehicle for experiencing this life. Infusing your body with energy and restoring your ability to move are essential for gaining the most out of physical existence.

- **You must move to escape CF/FMS.** Even if the extent of your ability is walking around the living room three times, do it regularly until you can do more. Work up gradually. A regular walk around the block is a goal to shoot for.

- **Give Qigong a try.** Possibly the best movement exercise for CF/FMS is the ancient Chinese art of Qigong (pronounced chi-gung). The slow, natural movements are easy to learn and provide a great way to restore balance in your energy pathways. A class with an instructor is ideal for learning Qigong but is not totally necessary. Qigong can be learned from a book, a DVD, or YouTube videos.

One of the easiest ways of learning basic Qigong is watching YouTube videos of people practicing Qigong. Some videos have been posted of people from Asian countries doing daily practice. The exercises are simple and easy to follow. Daily practice will dramatically decrease pain and increase mobility. If your interests progress beyond Qigong, you may decide to take up tai chi. Tai chi is actually just a complex form of Qigong.

- **Count your steps.** One of the best tools for increasing physical activity is a pedometer. A pedometer measures the steps you take. You can get a pedometer at any athletic store or from the Internet. Wear it every day. Initially, just record your baseline. As your health improves, try to increase daily steps. Your ultimate goal is 10,000 steps each day.

- **Warm up slowly.** Exercise moderately as long as it "feels good," and cool down adequately. If exercise results in a next-day hangover, with pain and increased fatigue, allow time to recover and back down on the level of intensity.

- **Don't overdo it.** Though exercise is beneficial, it is just as important not to overtax the body. Like hitting a wall, overdoing it can set you back a week or more. Learn your limits and gradually increase as the healing process allows.

- **Sign up for a yoga class.** Yoga is perfect for restoring your body. Basic yoga classifies as moderate physical activity; most anyone at any level of fitness and stamina can participate at some level. Classes are widely available in most every community. Even guys can benefit (no, you don't have to wear tights or act like a pretzel), but they probably will not be as flexible as female folk (or nearly as attractive doing yoga). Private lessons are worth considering for muscle stiffness and back pain. Yoga postures stretch ligaments and improve posture. Yoga encourages blood flow to areas of the body where flow can be restricted, such as the spine. Yoga is also a great way to generate endorphins.

- **Bounce back.** A rebounder is a small personal trampoline. If doing any sort of exercise is a challenge, a rebounder provides a safe and easy way to ease back in. Simply bouncing for 10–20 minutes a couple of times a day gets blood flowing, strengthens the autonomic nervous system, and increases lymphatic flow.[25]

- **Add some resistance.** Repetitions with light free weights systematically work the muscle groups of the body and are designed to increase muscle tone and physical strength. Resistance training is something that can wait until recovery is in full swing. Stay within your limits—"busting a gut" is not the goal.

- **Body rolling.** Body rolling is an interesting application of yoga poses using soft plastic balls to self-massage the spine and other parts of the body.

- **Work with a pro.** As your level of physical activity increases, you may find benefit from working with a personal trainer. A good personal trainer can help you reach a higher level of physical ability without risking injury. It is important to ask around and find someone who is sensitive to the issues of CF/FMS.

- **Make it fun.** As health improves, embracing an athletic activity can be very rewarding. Pick a low-intensity activity such as biking, hiking, golf, or kayaking.

- **Get outside.** Whenever weather allows, do something active outside. Strive for an hour each day! It's great for your vitamin D level and your outlook on life!

---

[25] rebound-uk.com/resourceArticles is a great resource for finding more information about the benefits of rebounding.

Movement is essential for overcoming CF/FMS, but movement is a stress on the body. Live life carefully. Think before you leap. Even minor trauma can set you back. All of the supplements recommended in this book for inflammation help reduce the damage caused by friction. Adaptogens, including rhodiola, cordyceps, and reishi, help you adapt to the physical stress of increased activity. Beyond the stress of being active, the physical stresses of pressure and temperature can also influence your recovery.

PRESSURE

High-pressure and low-pressure weather systems are always in motion across the face of the earth. While many people are unaffected by these minor changes in pressure, people with CF/FMS tend to be more sensitive. In general, high pressure is more comfortable and low pressure tends to make symptoms worse. Although there is nothing you can do about it, it is comforting to recognize why you may be feeling a little low yourself when a front passes through.

Pressure is also affected by change in elevation. Going abruptly from sea level to 8000 feet will very likely cause mild shortness of breath and mild exacerbation of symptoms. This should, however, resolve within a couple of days after you acclimate. The same thing can happen when traveling by air. Though the cabins in jetliners are pressurized, there is still an abrupt pressure change equivalent to 5000–7000 feet, and mild symptoms can occur. They should resolve when the plane lands, though you may feel "fuzzy" for a day or two after.

Altitude sickness

Decreased atmospheric pressure does not become a real problem until elevation crosses 8000 feet. At this elevation, pressure is low enough and the concentration of oxygen is thin enough that altitude sickness starts to become a concern. In general, people with

CF/FMS are more susceptible to altitude sickness than normal. Early symptoms of altitude sickness include shortness of breath, gasping, increased heart rate, palpitations, difficulty sleeping, slow mental function, extreme fatigue, nausea, and dizziness. It can progress to pulmonary edema (lungs filling with fluid), loss of consciousness, and even death. The treatment is going to a lower altitude as quickly as possible.

If you must go to a place with altitude greater than 8000 feet, go there slowly. Acclimate for a couple of days for every couple of thousand feet (if possible). If you begin having symptoms of altitude sickness, go back down and stay at that elevation until the symptoms resolve. You can then start back up, but very slowly.

Under the deep blue sea

Going in the opposite direction, the only natural way to decrease atmospheric pressure is by going under the surface of the sea. This concern, of course, is pertinent only to divers. Diving is a very reasonable activity for individuals with CF/FMS because it does not involve strenuous physical activity, but care should be taken not to overtax the body. Dive tables should be monitored carefully. Shallow dives and less stressful dives (short easy boat ride) are advisable until your health has been completely restored. Many divers report feeling better after diving if they use a special high-oxygen mixture called Nitrox. If you have never been diving and want to learn, it is advisable to wait until your recovery is well advanced.

TEMPERATURE

Winter can be a miserable time of year for people with CF/FMS. Cold hands, cold feet, and feeling chilled to the bone are a normal state much of the time. The metabolic fires are just not burning hot enough to keep everything warm. To recover from chronic fatigue, however, staying warm enough is really important. Fortunately, you do have some control.

- **Keep things warm.** Turn up the thermostat. Space heaters in offices, bedrooms, or other confined spaces can raise the temperature in the room without raising your heating bill significantly.

- **Layer.** Layer a sweater or vest over other clothes so you can easily adjust to temperature changes.

- **Take a warm bath.** When you feel your body getting chilled, a warm bath can do wonders.

- **Build a fire.** A fire in the fireplace (or woodstove) is also an excellent way to warm up a room on a cold winter day, but take special care that all toxins and smoke are well ventilated.

- **Try a sauna.** Sauna, especially FIR sauna, is a great way to warm, but be very careful to acclimate to higher temperatures very slowly. Excessive heat is just as stressful as excessive cold.

Though most CF/FMS patients prefer the heat of summer to the cold of winter, extreme heat can also be very debilitating. During the dog days of summer, an air conditioner is your best friend. Seek out shade and indoor environments during the middle of the day. Acclimate to hot outdoor conditions as slowly as possible.

Ambient temperatures over 90 degrees, especially if the humidity is high, should be avoided. This is especially true for exercising outdoors. Adequate hydration is essential, especially if you live in a dry climate. Signs of becoming overheated include loss of coordination, altered mental function, severe fatigue, nausea, dizziness, faintness, and increased heart rate. Sweating may or may not be present. Any of these signs should be taken as an indication to immediately get out of the heat and to hydrate with electrolyte/glucose-containing fluids.

For most people with CF/FMS, the most comfortable temperature range is 75–83 degrees Fahrenheit. One of the signs of improved health is being able to tolerate wider temperature variations, especially cooler temperatures.

When heat helps

Although oppressive heat can be extremely debilitating, brief exposure to heat under just the right circumstances can be comforting and restoring. FIR sauna and hot yoga are two examples of heat exposure that can relax stiff muscles and increase endorphins. Heat induces sweating, dilates blood vessels, and removes toxins. Warm up slowly and stop immediately if you feel uncomfortable.

- **Far infrared sauna (FIR).** FIR is an enclosed sauna using radiation to heat the body. Often referred to as "healing waves," far infrared radiation is at the opposite end of the spectrum from damaging gamma rays and x-rays. As the body is gently heated, toxins are pushed to the surface and released through sweat. The effectiveness and safety of FIR sauna is well documented in the scientific literature. FIR sauna has shown benefit for many types of chronic disease. Start with 10–20 minute sessions at a low temperature and work up to the recommended temperatures over several weeks. Discontinue if symptoms of CF/FMS are exacerbated.

- **Hot yoga.** This is a variation of yoga exercises performed in a hot environment. Temperatures vary from 85 to 110 degrees. Heat induces sweating, which removes toxins from the body. Heat also relaxes and soothes sore muscles. Many patients with fibromyalgia report decreased fatigue and pain with regular practice of hot yoga. Care, of course, must be taken not to get overheated. Start with brief exposure at lower temperatures. Stop the session if you start to feel bad; some days are going to be better than others. Never exceed more than an hour of exposure.

Four challenges down and four major attachments released into oblivion! If you've also been taking the supplements as recommended, your situation in life should be looking pretty good about now. If, however, you have only read the book and have not gotten started…what are you waiting for? A better life is just around the corner!

QUICK LIST

BASIC RECOVERY PROTOCOL

ESSENTIAL SUPPORT

General nutritional support

- **Multivitamin and mineral supplement.** Go beyond your average drugstore product. Look for products containing activated vitamins and minerals in organic form. Better products will have vitamin E in mixed tocopherol form instead of d-alpha tocopherol, methyltetrahydrofolate or folinic acid instead of folic acid, B12 as methylcobalimin or adenosylcobolimin, and minerals as amino acid chelates.

- **N-acetyl cysteine (NAC).** 1000–2000 mg twice daily.

- **Alpha lipoic acid.** 250–300 mg twice daily.

- **Milk thistle.** Dosage: 400–600 mg daily.

- **Vitamin C.** 500–1000 mg twice daily (higher dose is sometimes limited by the occurrence of loose stools).

- **Vitamin D.** Approximately 1000 IU daily (this amount is often found in multivitamin products), unless vitamin D levels suggest using higher amounts (discuss with your healthcare provider).

Reduction of inflammation

- **Resveratrol from Japanese knotweed.** Reduces tissue and vascular inflammation, improves blood flow. Protective of heart and nerve tissue.

  Dosage: See dosing below for antimicrobial benefit.

- **Combination anti-inflammatory supplement.** Look for one containing turmeric, boswellia, devil's claw, sea cucumber, glucosamine, and bromelain (or other enzyme). This combination can be found in various supplements and has been proven effective for reducing joint pain and inflammation.

  Dosage: Follow the dosage recommended on the supplement.

Immune support

- **Cordyceps.** Reduces inflammatory cytokine cascades, restores normal immune function. Adaptogenic—improves stress tolerance. Some antimicrobial properties. Protective of kidney function.

  Dosage: 1–3 grams (1000–3000 mg) cordyceps powder 2–3 times daily. (The higher dose range of 6–9 grams total per day is recommended during recovery.)

- **Reishi.** Reduces inflammatory cytokine cascades, restores normal immune function, has strong antiviral properties. Protective of liver function.

  Dosage: 1–2 grams (1000–2000 mg) standardized extract (10%–14% polysaccharides) twice daily. (Higher dose range of 4 grams daily recommended during recovery.)

- **Rhodiola.** Adaptogenic. Reduces fatigue, increases alertness. Antidepressant. Immune-modulating.

  Dosage: 100–200 mg of standardized extract (2%–3% rosavins, 0.8%–1% salidroside) twice daily.

- **Thymic extract.** Enhances immune function, increases T-cells and NK cells.

  Dosage: 1–3 packets of ProBoost daily until normal health is restored (for at least a month or two).

Antimicrobial support

- **Japanese knotweed.** Broad-spectrum antimicrobial against a wide range of bacteria, viruses, and fungi. Immune modulator.

  Dosage: 1–4 200 mg capsules Japanese knotweed (standardized to 50% trans-resveratrol) twice daily. Work up to 4 capsules twice daily and continue with that dosage until symptoms resolve. Once health is improved, gradually reduce to 1 capsule twice daily.

- **Chinese skullcap.** Potent synergist with strong antiviral properties and activity against mycoplasma.

  Dosage: 1 gram (1000 mg) 2–3 times daily. Use only the root extract, preferably 3-year plant with pronounced yellow color. (American skullcap does not offer the same antimicrobial properties and should not be substituted.)

Lyme disease spport

- **Eleuthero.** Improves resistance to stress (adaptogenic). Stimulates and moderates immune function. Antimicrobial properties.

  Dosage: 1:1 tincture (Russian extraction) from the root: 1 teaspoon twice daily (the second dose should be taken early in the afternoon to prevent evening stimulation). Dried herb extract: 500 mg twice daily. Extracts from the Siberian region of Russia or extracts grown in America are generally preferred to extracts obtained from China.

- **Cat's claw.** Primary herb for Lyme disease. Known to enhance a specific type of natural killer cell, called CD57, which is deficient in Lyme disease.

  Dosage: 1–4 400–500 mg capsules of 10:1 concentrate inner bark 2–3 times daily. Especially important to take this herb with food, as it is activated by stomach acid. If you take acid-blocking drugs, cat's claw will have limited value.

- **Andrographis.** Offers antiviral, antibacterial, and antiparasitic properties. Widely used in the treatment of Lyme disease.

  Dosage: 1–4 400 mg capsules, extract standardized to 10% andrographolides twice daily.

- **Sarsaparilla.** Binds endotoxins released from dying bacteria (reduces Herxheimer reactions). Potent synergist with other herbs. Antimicrobial properties.

  Dosage: 1–3 400–500 mg capsules of root extract twice daily.

- **Allisure garlic.** Patented extract of stabilized garlic. Broad-spectrum antimicrobial properties against bacteria, viruses, and yeast.

  Dosage: 180–360 mg 2–3 times daily.

SECONDARY SUPPORT

Stress

- **General stress.** Combination of Sensoril (patented ashwagandha), Relora (patented magnolia/philodendron species), and l-theanine is extremely effective for restoring balance in the face of stress. Balances the HPA axis, reduces anxiety, and improves sleep. Look for a combination supplement with these three ingredients, or take them each separately. All three are easy to find.

- **Anxiety/insomnia.** Often requires herbs with a stronger sedative effect. Bacopa, passionflower, and motherwort is a safe and proven combination.

- **Extreme fatigue with excessive sleepiness.** Requires stimulating herbs with adaptogenic properties. Panax ginseng, yerba mate, and guarana work well together—increases energy without causing excessive jitteriness.

Gastrointestinal support

- **Probiotic.** Include **lactobacillus** species and **bifidobacteria** species. Take 10–20 billion cfu twice daily.

- **Digestive enzymes.** Enhance digestion. Very important if gastrointestinal dysfunction is present.

Pain

- Talk to your healthcare provider about HCG or low-dose naltrexone for controlling pain.

LETTING GO OF SUPERFICIAL ATTACHMENTS

Attachment #1: commercially processed food
- Give up the bad stuff. Convenience and pacifying cravings are not worth the suffering.

- Enrich your life with vital energy from real food!

- Follow the recommendations in Chapter 7 to adapt your kitchen and palate to healthful eating.

Attachment #2: toxic lifestyle
- Cultivate toxin awareness.

- Follow the detoxification protocol at the end of Chapter 8.

Attachment #3: stressful lifestyle
- Let up on the pedal. Adrenaline and cortisol must be calmed throughout the day.

- Take a deep breath and say ohmmmmm. Practice relaxation exercises regularly!

- Strive for a good night's sleep—every night!

Attachment #4: inactivity

- Get out and do something—every day!

- Walking is a great place to start.

- Join a yoga class.

- If nothing else, get a rebounder and start bouncing!

Visit **rawlsmd.com** and **vitalplan.com** for updates and inspiration.

AFTERWORD

Atlantic Beach, North Carolina. Just to the left side of the fishing pier. Somewhere far offshore, a storm is pushing a light swell up onto the beach. Here, however, high pressure dominates; it couldn't be a more beautiful day. One of those rare late fall, early December days when the sky is clear and temperature hits 70. The sun is at its midday peak, and the air is perfectly still. Each wave is making a perfect curl as it encounters the slope of the shore. It is, in fact, a day almost exactly the same as the day seven years ago when I thought life was finished.

Except today, I'm catching almost every wave. No fatigue. No chest pain. No irregular heartbeats. I am surfing with a paddle board now; the paddle allows more oomph to get on the wave. Muscle strength is nowhere close to 100%; it probably never will be. Even so, I'm out here...and life isn't bad. There's no telling what tomorrow will bring, but I'll stay with the plan and take my supplements every day. Going about life in an easier manner has really been pleasant for a change.

I invite you to join me. The compromises to regain health have not really been compromises at all. Life is different—but better in so many ways.

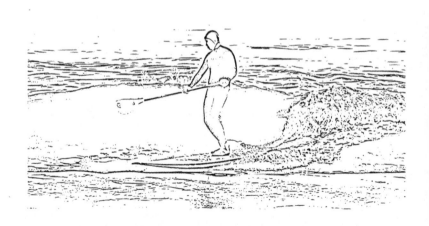

APPENDIX A

IMMUNE SYSTEM PRIMER

Of all the things that you must do to overcome CF/FMS, restoring normal immune function is the most important. Understanding the key players and pathways is useful for understanding chronic fatigue. The immune system can be divided into two major components: innate and adaptive. The innate immune system is nonspecific and targets any nonself threats. From an evolutionary point of view, the innate immune system is the most primitive and is the least complex. The adaptive portion of the immune system is very specific and has memory; in other words, it selects specific targets that it knows from past experience. The two systems can be defined as separate but are intimately connected and interdependent.

The innate immune system can be considered the outer wall of defense. It includes skin, hair in the nose, the mucosal lining of the intestinal tract, the lining of the lungs, and white blood cells (WBCs) that lie ready and waiting in those areas. The primary WBCs of the innate immune system, macrophages, attack anything foreign as soon as it steps foot in the door. They do not discriminate. They engulf the invader and place pieces of the invader on their surface (antigens) to act as a flag and send out messages to all other parts of the immune system (cytokines). Macrophages come in many varieties and are strategically placed at locations where foreign invaders can gain entrance.

Messages sent out by macrophages call in more specialized WBCs (neutrophils, eosinophils, basophils) to help deal with the threat. These are the classic inflammatory cells that secrete oxygen-generated free radicals, enzymes, hypochlorous acid, and other substances to destroy the offending substance or invader. An acute inflammatory reaction is a collection of these cells at the site of infection. Neutrophils are the most abundant and are important for destroying bacterial pathogens. Eosinophils target viruses and parasites. Basophils release histamine and are important for allergic reactions.

Another important cell type, natural killer (NK) cells are constantly on the prowl, searching for and destroying cells that have been stressed or that are infected by viruses or intracellular bacteria. NK cells are solitary soldiers that eliminate any cells that have lost the ability to look like "self." Elimination is not dependent on the abnormal cell being marked by antibodies; therefore, K cells can function independently of adaptive immunity. NK cells can be very important as a secondary backup when adaptive immunity has been compromised. Boosting NK cells is an important component of overcoming CF/FMS.

The second division of the immune system, adaptive immunity, constitutes the primary backup troops. These WBCs, called lymphocytes, are specialists. To function, they must have intelligence information and have a positive identification of the target. The first step in adaptive immunity is recognition of target. Macrophages (and dendritic cells, another type of "presenter" cell) present antigen (flag on the surface of the macrophage) from the engulfed threat to be "read" by circulating T-helper lymphocytes. If the body has been exposed to the threat before, an attack is immediately formulated. If the threat is new, it takes more time to educate all the troops, but a plan of attack still goes into motion. For a new threat that has never been recognized before, mobilizing the troops is typically a several-day affair.

There are two major divisions of the adaptive immune system. Cellular immunity comprises T-helper lymphocytes (CD4+), cells responsible for educating the troops, and cytotoxic T-lymphocytes (CD8+) that, once educated, recognize and destroy cells infected with intracellular pathogens or cells that are becoming cancerous. It is called cellular immunity because it deals only with abnormal cells that need to be eliminated. This is the arm of adaptive immunity that is involved with intracellular infections commonly associated with CF/FMS. Often, with CF/FMS, cellular immunity is overactive (which causes many of the symptoms) but dysfunctional at the same time. Not surprisingly, autoimmune disease is strongly linked to overactive cellular immunity. Cancer may also have links here as well.

Humoral immunity includes T-helper lymphocytes, which educate B-lymphocytes to recognize foreign antigens. B-lymphocytes produce antibodies against pathogens (viruses, bacteria, fungi, protozoa) that are present free and outside cells. Antibodies also target cellular debris and any other harmful materials. Antibodies can destroy the threat directly, mark the threat for engulfment by phagocytes (cells that engulf and digest the threat), or mark the threat for destruction by classic inflammatory cells (such as a worm too big to be engulfed). Different B-lymphocytes secrete different types of antibodies for different types of threats. This arm of adaptive immunity is often suppressed with CF/FMS.

Of course, all the soldiers in the system would be wandering around aimlessly without effective communication and direction. This is accomplished by an elaborate array of chemical messengers that circulate throughout the body. There are hundreds of different messengers, some that we know about, but probably many that are undiscovered (the complexity of the immune system is beyond imagination). The list includes cytokines (which send messages between lymphocytes) and chemokines (which call white blood cells to the area of infection). Low-virulence microbes have "learned" to manipulate cytokines to encourage destruction of tissues to gain access to valuable resources (different methods by different microbes). The flu-like symptoms associated with infection are actually caused by cytokines.

Association with autoimmune disease

Infection by a microbe that specializes in thriving inside cells compromises cellular immunity—the body loses the ability to destroy the microbes inside the cell. The microbe also blocks the ability of cytotoxic lymphocytes to destroy the abnormal infected cell. If these abnormal cells persist in the body, sooner or later, the second line of defense, humoral immunity, kicks in and antibodies are produced to eliminate the abnormal cells. These abnormal cells, however, still retain components of "self," and other normal cells get caught in the cross fire. Autoimmunity is the result of antibodies targeting normal cells in the body.

The process of autoimmunity can be quite persistent. Once a clone of antibody-producing B cells becomes active, antibodies will continue to be produced until the threat is long absent. Herbal therapies are beneficial for restoring normal cellular immunity, increasing NK cells (which act independently to eliminate abnormal cells), and eliminating the underlying threat. Herbs alone, however, will not suppress antibody production by B cells. It takes time for B-cell clones to become inactive and die off.

If the autoimmune process is severely destructive, steroid therapy is indicated. Steroids (prednisone, cortisone) dramatically suppress immune function across the board, including humoral immunity. This, of course, is a double-edged sword, because suppressing all immune function inhibits the ability of the immune system to overcome infections (of any type). Steroid therapy is sometimes indicated in the presence of a destructive autoimmune disease, but it should always be undertaken with great caution and always in conjunction with restoring herbal therapy.

APPENDIX B

EXTENDED SUPPLEMENT RECOMMENDATIONS

As stated previously, there are many natural supplement options for managing CF/FMS. The supplements discussed so far in the book are the primary supplements felt to offer the highest potential for benefit. One size, however, does not fit all. Certain people may not be able to tolerate one or some of the primary supplements, and people with more severe disease may need to take additional supplements; therefore, this list of alternative or additional supplements is provided.

PROTECT MITOCHONDRIA AND BOOST ENERGY

- **Glutathione.** Glutathione is an essential antioxidant inside cells for protecting mitochondria from free-radical damage during generation of energy. Glutathione is also essential for phase II detoxification in the liver. Glutathione is a large molecule composed of three amino acids, but intestinal absorption by oral administration of the reduced form has been documented. What is not known, however, is whether it crosses into cells and mitochondria from the bloodstream.

  Suggested dosage: 500–1000 mg twice daily of reduced glutathione.

  Side effects: Rare.

  At one point, I developed a pronounced head and hand tremor. It resolved completely within two weeks after I started 1000 mg of glutathione twice daily. The glutathione made me a believer, but right now, the stronger science is behind alpha lipoic acid and NAC. There is no harm in taking all three (except for the expense), but they perform similar functions; taking one of the three is satisfactory.

- **NADH (nicotinamide adenine dinucleotide).** NADH is an activated B vitamin important in energy production. Having a good supply present optimizes energy production in cells. Human studies have shown decreased fatigue in chronic fatigue with use of NADH.

  Suggested dosage: 10 mg twice daily. Sublingual dosing (under the tongue) may improve absorption.

  Side effects: Rare.

- **Lipid replacement therapy.** Mitochondria and cells are surrounded by a membrane made of special fats called phospholipids. Eggs, liver, beef brain, and soy are the highest natural sources of phospholipids, but there is some evidence that supplementing at higher levels than diet alone can improve everything from fatigue to cognitive function. The three main phospholipids—phosphatidylcholine (PC), phosphatidylserine (PS), and glycerophosphocholine (GPC)—are important for all cellular functions in the body, especially normal brain and muscle function.

  Suggested dosage: PC: 1–3 grams (1000–3000 mg) twice daily, PS: 200–500 mg twice daily, GPC: 200–300 mg twice daily. Ingredients can be obtained separately. Loose powder is the most cost effective and easily mixes with liquids. Dosage recommendations are purely an estimate based on studying products available and limited scientific studies available. Look for products free of GMO soy. (Taking these types of fats as part of your daily regimen can improve absorption of other supplements.)

  Side effects: None expected. Considered a functional food. Phospholipid supplements may actually enhance absorption of other supplements if taken together. Use with alpha lipoic acid (and/or glutathione), NAC, NADH, and CoQ10 for complete mitochondrial support.

Note that phospholipid supplements are bio-idenicals that have only a brief history of use and limited science for support. The potential for harm, however, is quite low. If you are interested, try them at the doses recommended for a 3-month period while holding all other supplements at constant doses. Monitor muscle strength, general fatigue, and post-exertion fatigue to decide whether you want to continue.

- **L-carnitine (acetyl-l-carnitine).** L-carnitine is important for metabolism of fatty acids in mitochondria. Has antioxidant properties. Protective of mitochondrial function. Acetyl-l-carnitine crosses the blood-brain barrier more effectively than does l-carnitine. Neuroprotective—can improve cognitive function.

  Suggested dosage: 500–1000 mg acetyl-l-carnitine twice daily.

  Side effects: none expected.

- **D-ribose.** A five-sided sugar (pentose) necessary for energy production. Though d-ribose supplements do not appear to improve strength or athletic performance, per se, they do appear to improve recovery. This is especially true in individuals with chronic fatigue or fibromyalgia. D-ribose can also reduce post-exertion pain.

  Suggested dosage: 1–3 grams (1000–3000 mg) twice daily (body builders use 5 grams three times daily). D-ribose is generally obtained as a powder with 1 teaspoon = 5 grams.

  Side effects: None expected. D-ribose is a natural sugar, but it does not raise insulin levels. It would take extremely large amounts daily to cause damage.

REDUCE INFLAMMATION

Tissue/Vascular inflammation

- **Rutin/Hesperidin.** Contains bio-flavonoid compounds known to increase integrity of blood vessels. Beneficial for the entire vascular system, but especially important for reducing risk of varicose veins. Also contains quercetin, a natural anti-histamine offering antimicrobial properties.

  Suggested dosage: 600–3000 mg combined daily.

  Side effects: Rare. Low potential for toxicity.

- **A rainbow of antioxidants.** Carotenoids are chemical compounds that provide yellow and red color in vegetables: the yellow in squash, the red in watermelon, and the orange in carrots. Another group of chemicals called anthocyanins provide the blue in berries. Carotenoids and anthocyanins are potent antioxidants offering protection to the skin, eyes, and vascular system. Your body cannot make these substances; they come only from fruits and vegetables...and though eating lots of fruit and vegetables is a great idea, adding on a supplement potentiates the benefit.

Joint and tissue inflammation

- **Collagen.** Natural collagen is beneficial for joints, ligaments, skin, hair, nails, and gums. Most products contain hydrolyzed collagen, low-molecular-weight hyaluronic acid, and chondroitin sulfate, the building blocks for new collagen. Several manufacturers (Biocell collagen, Neocell collagen), through a patented process, have been able to compact the molecular size of these substances for easy digestion and utilization by the body. Numerous human clinical trials document benefit, which includes strengthening and rebuilding of cartilage, ligaments, and joint structure, as well as replenishment of lubricating synovial fluid. Dosage depends on the product used.

- **Silicon.** Silicon is important for healthy bones, joints, hair, and nails. Silicon can be obtained from the herb horsetail, but possibly the best product is orthosilicic acid. Benefit from use of orthosilicic acid has been documented by clinical studies. Dosage depends on the product used.

- **SAMe.** SAMe is a molecule with anti-inflammatory properties. It enhances formation of molecules (proteoglycans) that pull water into cartilage. SAMe is also a mood elevator in individuals with depression. The incidence of side effects is low. SAMe should be avoided in individuals taking anti-depressant medications. Though efficacy for use of SAMe in arthritis is high, it is one of the most expensive supplements available.

  Suggested dosage: 600–1200 mg daily. Well tolerated.

- **MSM (methylsulfonylmethane).** MSM, given as a nutritional supplement, is converted into SAMe in the body. Less expensive than SAMe.

MICROBIAL SUPPORT

- **Anamu (Petiveria alliacea).** Anamu, an herb native to tropical regions of Central and South America, offers potent medicinal properties. Also known as guinea hen weed, anamu has been traditionally used for colds and flu, pain relief, pneumonia, and arthritis. Potent sulfur compounds give anamu a garlic-like odor. These and other chemical compounds offer potent broad-spectrum antimicrobial properties against bacteria, viruses, yeast, and fungi. Anamu is also immune-enhancing and offers potent anti-inflammatory properties (inhibits COX-1) and anticancer properties. It increases cellular immunity and increases NK cells. Anamu is known to provide activity against mycoplasma.

  Suggested dosage: 1–2 grams (1000–2000 mg) whole herb twice daily. Note that use of anamu will give urine and feces a distinct odor. Regular use will deter mosquito and tick bites.

Side effects: Safe and well tolerated. It should be avoided in pregnancy.

- **Artemisia (Artemisia annua).** Artemisinin, the primary chemical compound found in artemisia, is a potent antiparasitic (kills parasites) that is commonly used for treatment of malaria. Activity is primarily limited to blood parasites; general antibacterial activity is limited. Artemisia is primarily indicated when Babesia is suspected as a coinfection in Lyme disease.

  Suggested dosage: Depends on the preparation used. Artemisia should not be taken for longer than 7 days. Potency quickly declines with extended use. The dose can be repeated after 3 weeks.

  Side effects: Significant risk of neurotoxicity (damage to nervous tissue) with extended use.

OTHER NATURAL OPTIONS FOR PAIN

- **Corydalis yanhusua.** Corydalis[26] is a perennial herb in the poppy family native to Japan and Manchuria. The most commonly available species found in herbal supplements is corydalis. The medicinal value is derived from the rhizome (root). Traditionally, corydalis has been used for relief of menstrual cramps, relief of abdominal pain and cramps, and invigoration of the blood.

  Corydalis exhibits a strong analgesic effect (but is a hundred times less potent than morphine). It has a slower onset of action than morphine. Evidence of dependence has not been noted with corydalis. The herb has pronounced sedative qualities and improves sleep. It also has marked anti-inflammatory properties and improves coronary blood flow.

---

[26] My clinical experience with corydalis is limited. This information is derived from Chinese medical herbology and pharmacology.

Dosage: Approximately 1–1.5 grams (1000–1500 mg) dry powder 2–3 times daily. Dosage is highly dependent on the type of preparation used.

Side effects: Corydalis should not be used in pregnancy or with breast-feeding. Overdose can cause respiratory depression, sedation, and tremor.

ADDITIONAL OPTIONS FOR SLEEP

- **5-Hydroxy-tryptophan (5-HTP).** 5-HTP is a precursor for both serotonin and melatonin in the brain. During the day, it has a mood-stabilizing effect, and during the night, it can promote improved sleep. The recommended dose is 100 mg up to three times spread throughout the day or 100–300 mg at bedtime. 5-HTP is also metabolized as a normal substance in the body, and therefore, there is no risk of dependence or tolerance. Side effects are not common, but some patients report nightmares or muscle aches when using it regularly. The amino acid **tryptophan** can be substituted for **5-HTP.**[27]

- **Gamma amino butyric acid (GABA).** GABA is an important normal calming neurotransmitter in the brain. It is available as a supplement, but only a small amount of the supplemental dose crosses the blood-brain barrier. For some people, taking it as a supplement provides a mild sedative effect—for others, not so much. GABA should be used only intermittently because continual use suppresses normal GABA levels, which causes rebound insomnia to occur. Although it is mildly effective, continual use will suppress normal GABA in the brain and cause rebound insomnia to occur.

---

[27] Tryptophan and 5-HTP have been linked to a rare but life-threatening autoimmune condition called eosinophilia myalgia syndrome. In 1989, an outbreak of cases occurred, all commonly associated with supplementation with the amino acid tryptophan. The supplement was traced to a specific manufacturer in Japan. Whether the cause was tryptophan itself or an unknown contaminant (referred to as "peak X") has not been determined. The risk associated with pure forms of tryptophan and 5-HTP appears to be extremely low, but some caution is advised.

- **Glycine.** Glycine is an amino acid that provides a sedative effect when taken as a supplement. It acts very similarly to GABA and can cause rebound insomnia if taken continually. Use of glycine is very safe. The average dose is 1 g (1000 mg) at bedtime.

ADDITIONAL SUPPORT FOR THE GI TRACT

- **Cardamom.** Commonly used as a spice, cardamom is an excellent gastrointestinal tonic. Cardamom calms spasms in the stomach and intestines. It is great for stomachaches and gas pains. At the same time, cardamom improves gastric emptying and increases passage of food through the intestinal tract. It also provides a mild laxative effect.

  Suggested dosage: 300–500 mg taken up to 3–4 times daily.

  Side effects: Well tolerated. Should be avoided if gastric ulcers are present.

- **Demulcents.** These are substances that protect the stomach and intestinal lining and allow healing to occur. **Deglycyrrhizinated licorice (DGL)** is a special form of licorice that protects the lining of the gastrointestinal tract (non-stimulating and will not raise blood pressure). **Slippery elm** contains a substance called mucilage that protects the lining of the stomach and intestines. Good ole **Pepto Bismol** is great for settling stomach discomfort.

- **L-glutamine.** L-glutamine, an amino acid, is the primary energy source for intestinal cells. Supplementation with l-glutamine encourages healing in the GI tract. Average daily dose of glutamine in powder form is 1000–6000 mg, depending upon severity of disease.

ADAPTOGENS FOR SUPPORT OF PHYSICAL FITNESS

- **Rhaponticum carthamoides.** Rhaponticum is another Russian adaptogen with remarkable properties. Rhaponticum is anabolic, which means it builds lean muscle mass. Unlike anabolic steroids, however, it does not cause androgenic effects. Rhaponticum has caught the attention of many athletes, but it also offers characteristics that are beneficial for CF/FMS. It has been found to facilitate clearance of lactic acid (a toxic byproduct of metabolism) during exercise. Rhaponticum increases stamina and endurance. It balances the HPA axis and normalizes stressed adrenal function (normalizes cortisol). Sleep normalizes in stressed individuals. Rhaponticum is protective of heart and nerve function.

Rhaponticum was not chosen as a primary supplement because it is hard to find. About the only way to obtain it is as loose powdered extract or in athletic supplements that contain other undesirable ingredients. Also, it has not been extensively evaluated for immune-enhancing or antimicrobial properties.

Suggested dosage: 300–900 mg of standardized powdered whole plant or root extract (standardized to >5% ecdysterones).

Side effects: Unusual.

Future additions with be noted at rawlsmd.com

APPENDIX C

A VITAL-ENERGY GROCERY LIST

All natural foods are valuable, but certain functional foods offer exceptional levels of vital energy and promote healing. These foods should be included as regular staples.

- *Almonds.* Nuts in general are nutrient-dense nutrition sources, but almonds are especially good sources of calcium. (Be mindful of nut sensitivities.)

- *Asparagus.* This vegetable offers the highest natural known source of glutathione. Also contains histones that are felt to be important for decreasing cancer risk.

- *Avocado.* Avocados contain healthful monounsaturated fatty acids. Also a source of glutathione.

- *Berries.* Any berries, but especially blueberries, blackberries, and cherries, contain potent antioxidants. Tart cherries can improve sleep at night and reduce pain.

- *Brazil nuts.* Brazil nuts are a great source of selenium, which is very important for normal immune function. You don't want to overdo it, however; one or two a day is enough! (Be mindful of nut sensitivities.)

- *Carrots.* Carrots are a great source of carotenoids! The carotenoids lutein and zeaxanthin are potent antioxidants that build up in the skin and in the retina of the eyes, offering protection against the damaging effects of sunlight. All yellow vegetables offer lutein and zeaxanthin.

- *Celery.* Celery is mildly sedating and lowers blood pressure. It contains potent anticancer substances and will increase testosterone levels in men naturally.

- *Coconut oil.* The medium-chain saturated fatty acids found in coconut oil provide optimal fuel for energy production. Myristic acid and caprylic acid have some antimicrobial and antiyeast properties.

- *Cruciferous vegetables.* Broccoli, cabbage, cauliflower, kale, and other cruciferous vegetables are nutrient powerhouses. Kale is an especially good source of lutein.

- *Dandelion greens.* A mildly bitter green that is packed with nutrients including substantial amounts of vitamin C. Protective of liver function.

- *Eggs.* Low in calories and possibly the most cost-effective source of quality protein on the planet, eggs are also very nutrient dense. Phospholipids and choline, important for optimal health and normal brain function, are present in high concentrations in eggs. The yellow-orange color of egg yolk indicates carotenoids, and eggs are another great source of these important antioxidants. Local farm eggs contain higher concentrations of nutrients and lower levels of cholesterol than the grocery-store variety.

- *Ginger.* The potent anti-inflammatory substances found in ginger reduce inflammation in the body but are especially beneficial for healing inflammation in the stomach and intestines. Ginger is also a potent antiviral if used fresh as a strong tea.

- *Melons.* Melons are a good source of superoxide dismutase and glutathione (important cellular antioxidants). Watermelons are a great source of lycopene, a potent antioxidant important for prostate health. And, of course, watermelons provide lots of water!

- *Mushrooms.* A low-calorie and flavorful addition to any dish, mushrooms are a good source of B vitamins, minerals, and vitamin D. Many types of mushrooms boost immune function, and some may reduce cancer risk. Don't be afraid to venture past common white mushrooms and try other varieties.

Portabella, brown button, shiitake, maitake, and oyster have slightly different flavors.

- *Olive oil.* Olive oil is one of the best sources of monounsaturated fatty acids. Also, substances in olive oil offer antimicrobial properties.

- *Onions.* Besides tasting great, onions and garlic nurture friendly bacteria in the gut and provide antibiotic properties against pathogenic bacteria. Eat onions every day!

- *Oysters.* Besides being very tasty, oysters are a great source of zinc and other important nutrients.

- *Pomegranate juice.* Pomegranate seeds and juice contain potent antioxidants and also offer antimicrobial properties.

- *Pumpkin seeds.* Raw or roasted pumpkin seeds provide a great tree-nut alternative for individuals with nut sensitivities. The oils in pumpkin seeds support prostate health.

- *Sesame oil.* Sesame seeds are another great source of monounsaturated fatty acids. Tahini, a paste made from sesame seeds, is a component of hummus.

- *Sea vegetables.* Seaweeds are excellent natural sources of iodine, important for normal thyroid function. Iodine levels in sea vegetables are, however, highly variable. Talk to your healthcare provider about consuming sea vegetables regularly if you have a thyroid disorder.

- *Spirulina.* Spirulina is a nutrient-dense sea vegetable that is a complete source of protein.

- *Sunflower seeds.* A great tree-nut alternative that can be consumed by individuals with tree-nut allergies or sensitivities. Sunflower butter is a great alternative to peanut butter.

- *Vinegar.* The acetic acid in vinegar improves digestion and activates digestive enzymes. Vinegar is known to improve calcium absorption and to support healthy bones. Vinegar also improves glucose metabolism and reduces risk of diabetes. Apple cider vinegar can be taken as a daily health supplement, 2 tablespoons in 6 oz. of water with each meal.

- *Walnuts.* Walnuts are a great source of healthful fats, fiber, and glutathione. (Be mindful of nut sensitivities.)

REFERENCES
AND READING LIST

No list is totally inclusive. Much of knowledge is derived from experiencing life. Personal experience with CF/FMS provided me with knowledge that could not have been gained any other way. Working directly with patients each day and using natural supplements in clinical practice has provided me a wealth of knowledge that cannot be documented. General knowledge from the Internet, including product information provided by supplement companies and testimonials, also has great value.

The ability to share information is one of the most extraordinary miracles of our time. I and the world owe a great debt to the individuals in the references below who took their time to share hard-won experience and expertise with the rest of the world.

The ABC Clinical Guide to Herbs
Mark Blumenthal, Editor
American Botanical Council, Copyright 2003
ISBN 1-58890-157-2

Adaptogens: Herbs for Strength, Stamina, and Stress Relief
David Winston and Steven Maimes
Healing Arts Press, Copyright 2007
ISBN 978-1-59477

Adaptogens in Medical Herbalism
Donald Yance Jr., CN, MH, RH(AHG)
Healing Arts Press, Copyright 2013
ISBN 978-1-62055-100-4

Advanced Nutrition and Human Metabolism, 3rd Edition
James L. Groff, Sareen S. Gropper
Wadsworth, Copyright 2000
ISBN 0-534-55521-7

Allicin: The Heart of Garlic
Peter Josling
HRC Publishing, Copyright 2005
ISBN 1-900052-10-5

Ayurvedic Medicine: The Principles and Traditional Practice
Sebastian Pole
Churchill Livingstone/Elsevier, Copyright 2006
ISBN 978-0-443-10090-1

Basic Immunology
Abul K. Abbas, MBBS, and Andrew H. Lichtman, MD, PhD
Saunders/Elsevier, Copyright 2011
ISBN 978-1-4160-5569-3

The Blue Zones, 2nd Edition
Dan Buettner
National Geographic Society, Copyright 2012
eISBN 978-1-4262-0949-9

Chinese Medical Herbology and Pharmacology
John K. Chen and Tina T. Chen
Art of Medicine Press, Copyright 2001
ISBN 0-9740635-0-9

Foods That Fight Pain
Neal Barnard, MD
Three Rivers Press, Copyright 1998
ISBN 0-609-80436-7

Harper's Biochemistry, 25th Edition (a large medical book)
Robert K. Murray, MD, PhD; Daryl K. Granner, MD; Peter D.
Mayes, PhD, DSC; Victor W. Rodwell, PhD
McGraw-Hill, Copyright 2000
ISBN 0-8385-3684-0

Healing Lyme Disease Coinfections
Stephen Harrod Buhner
Healing Arts Press, Copyright 2013
ISBN 978-1-62055-008-3

*Healing Lyme: Natural Healing and Prevention of Lyme Borre-
liosis and Its Coinfections*
Stephen Harrod Buhner
Raven Press, Copyright 2005
ISBN 978-0-9708696-3-0

The Healing Power of Rainforest Herbs
Leslie Taylor, ND
Square One Publishers, Copyright 2005
ISBN 0-7570-0144-0

Herbal Antibiotics
Stephen Harrod Buhner
Storey Publishing, Copyright 2012
ISBN 978-1-60342-987-0

Herbal Antivirals
Stephen Harrod Buhner
Storey Publishing, Copyright 2013
ISBN 978-1-61212-160-4

Herbal Medicine, Healing and Cancer
Donald Yance Jr., CN, MH, AHG
McGraw-Hill, Copyright 1999
ISBN 978-0-87983-968-0

Herbal Therapy & Supplements, 2nd Edition
Merrily A. Kuhn and David Winston
Wolters Kluwer Health/Lippincott Williams & Wilkins, Copyright 2008
ISBN 978-1-58255-462-4

Hyperhealth Pro Version 10—extensive database on health resources and natural ingredients

Iceman Autopsy
Stephan S. Hall
National Geographic magazine
November 2011

Living Well with Hypothyroidism
Mary J. Shomon
Harper Resource, Copyright 2005
ISBN 0-06-074095-7

The Lyme Disease Solution
Kenneth B. Singleton, MD, MPH
Brown Books, Copyright 2008
ISBN-13: 978-1-934812-00-6

Medical Herbalism: The Science and Practice of Herbal Medicine
David Hoffmann, FNIMH, AHG
Healing Arts Press, Copyright 2003
ISBN 978-089281749-8

Medical Microbiology, 24th Edition
Geo F. Brooks, MD; Karen C. Carroll, MD; Janet S. Butel, PhD; Stephen A. Morse, PhD
Lange/McGraw-Hill, Copyright 2007
ISBN 978-0-07-147666-9

Medicines from the Earth (lecture notes)
Conference May 31–June 4, 2013
Annual conference on herbal medicine
Black Mountain, NC

The Menopause Thyroid Solution
Mary J. Shomon
HarperCollins, Copyright 2009
ISBN 978-0-189897-6

Modern Nutrition Health and Disease, 9th Edition
Donna Bulado, Editor
Williams and Wilkins, Copyright 1999
ISBN 0-683-30769-X

Mortalility by Neoplasia and Cellular Telephone Base Stations
in the Belo Horizonte Municipality, Minus Gerais State, Brazil
Adilza C. Dode et al.
Science of the Total Environment
May 2011
Elsevier

The Okinawa Program
Bradley J. Willcox, MD; D. Craig Willcox, PhD; Makoto Suzuki,
MD
Three Rivers Press/Random House, Copyright 2001
ISBN 0-609-80750-1

PDR for Herbal Medicines, 1st Edition
Medical Economics Company, Copyright 1998
ISBN 1-56363-292-6

PDR for Nutritional Supplements, 2nd Edition
Sheldon Saul Hendler, PhD, MD, FACP, FACN, FAIC
Thomson Reuters, Copyright 2008
ISBN 978-1-56363-710-0

The Relaxation and Stress Reduction Workbook, 5th Edition
Martha Davis, PhD; Elizabeth Robbins Eshelman, MSW;
Matthew McKay, PhD
New Harbinger Publications, Inc., Copyright 2000
ISBN 1-57224-214-0

Review of Medical Microbiology and Immunology
Warren Levinson, MD, PhD
Lange/McGraw-Hill, Copyright 2012
ISBN 978-0-07-177433-8

Review of Medical Physiology, 20th Edition (a large medical
book)
William F. Ganong, MD
McGraw-Hill, Copyright 1999
ISBN 0-8385-8282-6

Website references

naturaldatabase.com—Paid resource for scientific data about
nutraceuticals. Evidence-based.

naturalstandard.com—Paid resource for scientific data about
nutraceuticals. Evidence-based.

herbalgram.org—American Botanical Council website provides extensive research and information about the clinical
use of herbal therapy. Membership required. Evidence-based.

eatwild.com—Resource for finding naturally produced meat
in your area.

ewg.org—Environmental Working Group is a nonprofit orga-
nization dedicated to providing information about living a
healthful lifestyle.

rawlsmd.com—For updates, recipes and further information.

vitalplan.com—Information about natural supplements and
healthful living.

ACKNOWLEDGEMENTS

First and foremost, I would like to thank my patients, who over the years have taught me much. I would especially like to thank individual patients, Judy Wooten, Debra Stinson, Jeanine Early, Deborah Frisby, Cathy Adair, Joy Velasquez, Clemma Florio, and Marion Morris, who read early versions of the book and gave essential feedback. Without their input, the book would not have had true value.

A special thanks to Courtney Wilson, FNP, for her professional expertise and feedback on the book.

Also special thanks to Christie Fulcher, RN and Patty Boone at my office for all of their help along the way.

I would like to thank Paula Ford-Martin at Workcrafts, for her profession editing and direction in making the book more readable and user friendly.   I would also like to thank Jennifer, associated with Dog Ear publishing, for her excellent job at copy editing.

Thanks to everyone at Dog Ear publishing for putting up with my obsessive-compulsive behavior in getting the book just right.

Thanks to Braden and Esther at Vital Plan for helping with ideas and giving feedback.

Thanks especially to my wife, Meg, for putting up with the arduous book writing process and always being there to bounce ideas and opinions off it.

PERSONAL BIO

Dr. Rawls attended medical school at Wake Forest University. He is board certified in obstetrics and gynecology and maintains a license to practice medicine in the state of North Carolina. Formal professional training is complemented by a passion for the study of concepts in natural medicine. Ten years of intensive self-study in herbal medicine and other natural therapies combined with numerous seminars and a certification course in holistic medicine define his present practice focused on health restoration.

Dr. Rawls resides on the coast of North Carolina, where he enjoys other passions, including boating, kayaking, kitesurfing, and yoga. He lives with his wife of thirty years, who teaches biology at a local community college. Together, they live and promote concepts of wellness. Their two adult children are also involved in health-and-wellness professions.

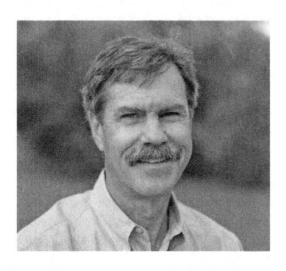

Index

CPSIA information can be obtained
at www.ICGtesting.com
Printed in the USA
BVOW06s1143261116

468717BV00007B/107/P